Fetal Heart Ultrasound

We only find what we look for

We only look for what we know

We only know what we understand

Associate Editor: Dinah Thom
Project Manager: Emma Riley
Designer: Stewart Larking
Illustration Manager: Bruce Hogarth
Multimedia Production Manager: Colin McEwan
Illustrator: Jane Fallows based on original drawings by Loic Fredouille and Alexandre Fleury
Histological sections: Maxette Pierrin and Pascal Blain
DVD compiler: Pascal Blain

Fetal Heart Ultrasound

How, Why and When

3 Steps and 10 Key Points

Catherine Fredouille MD

Part-time Hospital Practitioner, Fetal Placentology Unit, Hôpital de La Timone, Marseilles, and Consultant in Fetopathology, Department of Cytogenetics and Fetopathology, Hôpital Armand-Trousseau, Paris, France

Jean-Eric Develay-Morice MD

Nîmes Maternity Service, Hôpital Carrémeau, Nîmes, France

Translated by
Sheldon Heitner

With forewords by
Professor Antoine Casasoprana
Honorary Professor in Paris VII-Lariboisière University, and formerly Chief of the Cardiopediatric Unit, Hôpital R. Debré, Paris, France

Professor Pierre Mares
Nîmes Maternity Service, Hôpital Carrémeau, Nîmes, France

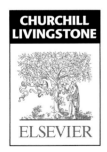

CHURCHILL
LIVINGSTONE

ELSEVIER

EDINBURGH   LONDON   NEW YORK   OXFORD   PHILADELPHIA   ST LOUIS   SYDNEY   TORONTO   2007

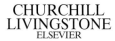

CHURCHILL
LIVINGSTONE
ELSEVIER

An imprint of Elsevier Limited

First edition published in French under the title *Cœur fœtal pratique: 3 temps – 10 points-clés*
© 2003, Sauramps Médical

First edition published in English
© 2007, Elsevier Limited. All rights reserved.

First edition 2003
English edition 2007
  Reprinted 2008

ISBN 978-0-443-10332-2

British Library Cataloguing in Publication Data
A catalogue record for this book is available from the British Library

Library of Congress Cataloging in Publication Data
A catalog record for this book is available from the Library of Congress

Notice
Knowledge and best practice in this field are constantly changing. As new research and
experience broaden our knowledge, changes in practice, treatment and drug therapy may
become necessary or appropriate. Readers are advised to check the most current information
provided (i) on procedures featured or (ii) by the manufacturer of each product to be
administered, to verify the recommended dose or formula, the method and duration of
administration, and contraindications. It is the responsibility of the practitioner, relying on
their own experience and knowledge of the patient, to make diagnoses, to determine
dosages and the best treatment for each individual patient, and to take all appropriate safety
precautions. To the fullest extent of the law, neither the publisher nor the authors assume
any liability for any injury and/or damage to persons or property arising out or related to
any use of the material contained in this book.

The Publisher

Working together to grow
libraries in developing countries

www.elsevier.com | www.bookaid.org | www.sabre.org

ELSEVIER | BOOK AID International | Sabre Foundation

ELSEVIER your source for books,
journals and multimedia
in the health sciences
www.elsevierhealth.com

The
publisher's
policy is to use
**paper manufactured
from sustainable forests**

Printed in China

Contents

DVD Contents

This first section which lasts 27 minutes is dedicated to a demonstration of the normal anatomy of the fetal heart on anatomical specimens.

The anatomical description of the Position, including the abdominal situs and the position of the organs as well as the position of the vessels, is followed by a "guided" tour of the fetal heart.

First, the **External guided tour** shows the systemic and pulmonary venous return, the atria and appendages, the ventricles and then, the great vessels: the pulmonary trunk, its branches and the ductus and the aorta.

An **Internal guided tour** leads you inside a normal fetal heart. First, we visit the right tract:

– The right atrium with its pectinate muscles, the Eustachian and Thebesian valves, the foramen ovale and its flap valve
– The right atrioventricular valve is the tricuspid valve with its three leaflets
– The right ventricle with inlet, apical trabecular and outlet with the pulmonary arterial trunk.

Then, the left tract with:

– The left atrium
– The left atrioventricular valve which is the mitral valve and its two leaflets
– The left ventricle with inlet, apical trabecular, outlet.

We'll finally emphasize the differences between inlet and outlet and the alignment and misalignment of the aorta.

We show on anatomical specimens the location of the main ultrasonographical incidences.

First of all, the **"Optimal" fetal four-chamber view** and its hallmarks. On this view, we show the descending aorta, the left atrium, the inferior vena cava and the foramen ovale. We describe the atrioventricular concordance and the axis of the heart. Finally, we zoom in on the crux of the heart.

The second view described is the **Long axis left outflow plane.**

Then, the **Three-vessel view.** Finally, we show the **ductus arteriosus plane.** We insist on **the importance of the infundibulum in the CT spectrum.**

This section shows, without sound, the ultrasound images depending on the use of different settings:

Zoom: when not enough zoom is used or when it is well adapted. There follows a description of the maximal zoom necessary to emphasize the crux of the heart.

Focus: can be too high or correct.

Gain: is often too high or too low. It has to be in a correct setting.

In case Doppler is used, the **Size of the box,** the **Angle of incidence** and the **PRF** are of great importance.

There are **Other 2D settings** such as **Dynamic range, Persistence, Contours, Frequency, Density of lines, Post-treatment G and Delta.**

3. METHODOLOGY   (20 MIN)

The first part of this section of 20 min is with sound. It demonstrates our methodology.

Comparing the US fetal heart examination to the **Reading of a book,** we first explain the use of the **Situs Wheel.** Then, we describe the different steps and elements of our methodology based on **Fetal pathological correlations:**

– the "elevator"
– the TAD four-chamber view translation
– the Reference points of the four-chamber view
– the Quality criteria of the "optimal" four-chamber view
– the Situation of the great vessels.

The second part, without sound, shows the **Application of our methodology to the echographic fetal heart examination:**

After US images of the translation with the **Elevator to the Four-chamber view,** we insist on the **reference points of the "optimal" four chamber view:** apex and two pulmonary veins. After the explanation of the **Axis of the heart** and the search for the **Aorta on the left,** there is a demonstration of what **2D and color fast glances** show. Back to the **"optimal" four-chamber view,** there are answers to the questions: **Where and How?**

The **LV-Ao,** the **RVPT,** the **Three-vessel view,** the **Aortic arch view** and **Ductus arteriosus view** are shown in the same way.

4. PITFALLS (WITH SOUND)   (3 MIN)

This short sequence shows how the "optimal" four-chamber view can be misinterpreted in case of a **Lateral, Inferior** or **Superior swing.**

5. PATHOLOGIES (WITH SOUND)
(28 MIN)

This section, which shows anatomical and echographical images of pathologies, follows the same order as the book.

First the **Pathologies of position** with the viscero-atrial heterotaxias (VAH).

The anomalous systemic venous return with a lack of inferior vena cava and azygos venous return in case of left isomerism is shown before an anomalous pulmonary venous return in case of right isomerism. Then, we describe the cardiac pathologies encountered in VAH.

In the **Pathologies seen in the inlet,** after a description of total anomalous pulmonary venous return (TAPVR), a large part is dedicated to all the pathologies of the AVSD spectrum. After an Introduction, the different forms of the AVSD spectrum are explained: complete AVSD, partial AVSD, and the newly described linear insertion of the atrioventricular valves (LIAVV) without defect.

Then we describe a quite difficult pitfall consisting of a dilated coronary sinus associated with a minor hypoplastic left heart syndrome (HLHS) and an aortic bicuspidia.

Also diagnosed in the inlet, the HLHS and its spectrum occurs more often than right ventricular hypoplasia (RVH).

In the **Pathologies seen in the outlet,** the most important in prenatal diagnosis is the complete transposition of the great vessels (TGV).

Often associated with other pathologies, we insist on the conotruncal cardiopathy (CTC) spectrum. After an Introduction, we give examples of the asymmetry of the vessels in a tetralogy of Fallot (ToF) and an interruption of the aortic arch (IAA).

We show the constant ventricular septal defect (VSD) and on the CTC hallmarks possibly seen in the inlet.

A detailed description of the pathologies of the conotruncal spectrum follows depending on the swing of the infundibulum : anterior in ToF and pulmonary atresia with opened septum (PAOS), the agenesis of the pulmonary valves being a particular case. It is a posterior swing which is responsible for the IAA interruption of the aortic arch we describe in "B".

We conclude this chapter about CTC hallmarks which must not be missed such as: right aorta and 60° axis; LIAVV in the four-chamber view; large aorta.

Foreword

Antoine Casasoprana

Fetal ultrasound is a young technique. Apart from early pioneering experiments, it is not yet 30 years old. At the beginning of the 1980s in the maternity ward of the Hôpital Saint-Maurice, France, François Éboué did his best to reconstruct cardiac structures and fetal vasculature using the pale sweep of the TM mode; we can remember his passionate commentaries as he showed us poorly contrasted two-dimensional images. In 1984 Laurent Fermont returned from Montreal where he had been trained under Jean-Claude Fouron and began practicing prenatal ultrasound in Paris, at much the same time as Bernard de Geeter in Strasbourg. Others followed, after they had qualified in pediatric cardiology, obstetrics, gynecology, or radiology.

However, for many practitioners, even those specializing in fetal ultrasound, examination of the fetal heart continued to live up to its reputation of being extremely difficult. This is for several reasons: the transversal position of the fetal heart in the thorax; the difficulty involved in defining situs in the presentation of the fetus; and, above all, to the rolling and twisting of the ventricular exit pathways and of the two great vessels, with a ductal arch next to the aortic arch. The authors of this book dedicate a large part of their work to explaining this embryology through the use of fetal pathological images, thus helping us to understand the situation better, as well as illustrating their points.

The discovery of a prenatal cardiac anomaly necessitates critical investigation of other pathologies, which, in turn, could perhaps reveal a syndrome, with all the ethical problems and serious decisions that this type of discovery implies. An important part of this book is dedicated to this difficult problem.

Catherine Fredouille has two of the qualities needed to be a good teacher. First, she practices the science she teaches, carrying out ongoing research to remain at the cutting edge of our understanding of fetal pathology. Second, she knows how to translate what she has learned into a didactic and often playful style of teaching, taking such pleasure in transmitting this knowledge that she creates the same response in her audience. With Jean-Eric Develay-Morice she has produced a useful book, very much orientated towards practice. I wish them success, and predict that this book will be of great benefit to all ultrasound specialists who perform this difficult prenatal examination.

Foreword

Pierre Mares

The fetal heart seen through ultrasound… from the symbolic to the digital image! Studying the fetal heart represents a medical challenge of the highest order for the future of the fetus. Considered for a long time as being at the very technical limits of ultrasound itself, today its use in the analysis of cardiac architecture has become a new paradigm.

It requires flawless equipment as well as a competent operator with a thorough knowledge of embryology, anatomy, and hemodynamics. The difficulty in analyzing cardiac structure is often linked to a lack of knowledge in one of these crucial fields.

Catherine Fredouille and Jean-Eric Develay-Morice bring their experience to bear in ultrasound with an in-depth analysis of fetal pathology, offering us a remarkable work which integrates the three aspects of embryology, anatomy, and hemodynamics.

They lead us successively through a series of illustrations outlining embryology and cardiac anatomy. They explain and justify the planes and sections necessary to study the zones of the heart, especially anomalies that up to now have not been well documented but may be suspected, as soon as the reference image of normality is not acquired or seen.

When approached from this standpoint the fetus presenting with a cardiac malformation will be detected and then analyzed at an anatomic level, thus benefiting from the latest and most up-to-date medical expertise.

Scholastically remarkable as well as open to the latest research, this book is recommended to all those interested in detecting cardiac malformations in particular and prenatal diagnosis in general.

Acknowledgments

With thanks to:

Professors J. F. Pellissier, D. Figarella-Branger, P. Mares, J.-L. Taillemite, and J.-P. Siffroi;

the members of the Société Française d'Imagerie en Gynécologie et Obstétrique (SFIGO; the French Society for Ultrasound in Gynecology and Obstetrics) and the Collège Français d'Échographie Fœtale (CFEF; the French College for Fetal Ultrasound)

who participated in the "4 Chambers" and "Crux of Heart" protocols;

all those who allowed us the use of their images: Doctors M. Althuser, P. Bailleul, N. Bigi, N. Fries, J. C. Gicquel, and D. Le Duff;

our "supporters": Doctors M. Gonzales, Y. Huten, C. Talmant, and M. Yvinec; and

our friends at the CFEF.

Abbreviations

22q1.1 del	deletion of the 22nd chromosome in q1.1	IVS	interventricular septum
AD	arterial duct (= ductus arteriosus)	LA	left atrium
Ao	aorta	LAp	left appendage
AR	autosomal recessive	LCA	left carotid artery
ASD	atrial–septal defect	LIAVV	linear insertion of atrioventricular valves
AVC	atrioventricular canal	LIPV	left inferior pulmonary vein
AVSD	atrioventricular septal defect	LPA	left pulmonary artery
AVV	atrioventricular valves	LPVC	left persistent vena cava
CAT	common arterial trunk	LSCA	left subclavian artery
CHD	congenital heart disease	LV	left ventricle
CRL	cranial rump length	MAPCA	main aorta–pulmonary collateral arteries
CTC	conotruncal cardiopathy	MS	membranous septum
CS	coronary sinus	MTP	medical termination of pregnancy
DA	ductus arteriosus (= arterial duct)	NT	nuchal translucency
dB	decibel	PA	pulmonary atresia
Es	esophagus	PA with IS	pulmonary atresia with intact septum
FNB	fetal nasal bone	PA with OS	pulmonary atresia with opened septum
FO	foramen ovale		
FOV	foramen ovale valve	PRF	pulse repetition frequency
HLB	heart–lung block	PT	pulmonary trunk
HLHS	hypoplastic left heart syndrome	PV	pulmonary vein
HLV	hypoplastic left ventricle	PVR	pulmonary venous return
HRV	hypoplastic right ventricle	RA	right atrium
IAA	interruption of the aortic arch	RAp	right appendage
IAS	interatrial septum	RCA	right carotid artery
IURG	intrauterine retarded growth	RIPV	right inferior pulmonary vein
IVC	inferior vena cava		

ROSCA	retro-esophagal subclavian artery	TAD	transabdominal diameter
RPA	right pulmonary artery	TAPVR	total anomalous pulmonary venous return
RSCA	right subclavian artery		
RV	right ventricle	TGV	transposition of the great vessels
SLOS	Smith–Lemli–Opitz syndrome	ToF	tetralogy of Fallot
STIC	spatiotemporal image correlation	UA	unique atrium
SVC	superior vena cava	UUA	unique umbilical artery
SVR	systemic venous return	US	ultrasound
T	trachea	UV	unique ventricle
T13	trisomy 13 (Patau's syndrome)	VAH	visceroatrial heterotaxia
T18	trisomy 18 (Edwards' syndrome)	VSD	ventricular septal defect
T21	trisomy 21 (Down's syndrome)		

Chapter 1

Why: fetal heart ultrasound

by Catherine Fredouille

 This chapter is also covered in Part 1 of the accompanying DVD

The heart examination is a critical moment in fetal ultrasound (US). After birth cardiologists carry out this examination, but before then the fetal heart is seen by non-cardiologists. While it is not necessary to have the level of knowledge of a pediatric cardiologist to perform this systematic prenatal check-up, it is essential to acquire a simple, solid knowledge base if we are to carry out fetal heart examinations that are valid and have a long-term prognostic value.[1] This can only contribute to the development of our specialty.[2]

We hope that this will be the sort of book that we would have wanted to find years ago when we began studying fetal hearts. There have always been excellent "classical" reference books which teach pediatric cardiology as applied to the fetus. They contain much more than what is needed in our daily practice, and because of this, require long and attentive research to find the answers essential to fetal US. What we are trying to do here is provide a practical guide for the US practitioner, underlining the elements that we have found through our experience to be essential.

We are both practicing fetal US specialists, each with different but constantly evolving and complementary interests and skills. Jean-Eric Develay-Morice is more involved in the technical aspects of our craft, specifically concentrating on finding new ways to diagnose previously "undiagnosable" pathologies.

I have spent the last several years in the anatomic examination of thousands of fetal hearts, normal as well as pathological, using a strict segmental analysis.

I then apply this work to US–anatomic correlations. Over the years of close collaboration, we found that, above all, the US specialist needed tools to test for what we call "normality".

Our experience has shown that the pathologies involved in the fetuses with the worst prognosis were always of the same type. We learned that what is "essential" is to be able to say that a fetal heart looks normal by checking for simple warning signs, rather than being able to precisely diagnose all types of pathologies. This is seen to be true in a great majority of cases.

When faced with a cardiopathy, the role of the practitioner is to ensure that there is not an associated extracardiac pathology. The warning signs we propose are simple, and we explain how to check for them. We do this using visual comparisons, which come from our experience teaching in tandem during numerous workshops in France and the Mediterranean region. We kept what worked best in our original French edition, the same style, and the same conscious insistence on repetition.

Repetition has proved to be an essential part of our methodology, providing a book that is fundamental and practical for daily use. To increase its value as a training and reference tool, we have added references and a DVD, which includes US sequences, a large section on anatomy with a guided tour—inside and out—of the fetal heart, and another section underlining anatomic and US correlations. We hope that you will find in this book and its DVD practical keys to the practice of fetal heart US.

One of our primary intentions is to introduce information which is indispensable for verifying normal fetal heart architecture, as well as information useful in the detection of important pathologies. The precise diagnosis of cardiopathies, and their prognoses, remains the realm of the pediatric cardiologist.

The US practitioner has several aims. One is to verify normal fetal cardiac architecture, which also involves looking for cardiopathies in the case where another anomaly has presented itself during morphological examination. It can also involve the discovery of an isolated cardiopathy, but this is a rare event.

Here we will lay out a simple methodology capable of verifying normal fetal cardiac architecture in 3 steps and 10 key points rather than a compre-

hensive or exhaustive screening.[3] These key points have been defined through a series of anatomic–US correlations and tested by numerous US specialists. The diagnostic criteria are easily accessible and allow us to eliminate important cardiopathies detectable in the fetus.

We begin by reviewing the knowledge essential in understanding what is normal, as well as pathologic, in the fetal heart. We then touch on those physical principles crucial in optimizing the examination itself, finally introducing our methodology. Next, we study the pathologies themselves, outlining the pitfalls involved in studying each one while proposing the best methods for avoiding these traps. Finally, we will describe the type of morphological examination necessary in those cases where a cardiopathy has been discovered, concluding with a review of points to remember.

GENERAL NOTIONS

In the fetus there are two types of cardiopathies that are important to detect:

- Cardiopathies that are warning signs of chromosomal anomalies, syndromes or associations. Our own fetal pathologic experience, as well as that of other teams,[4] has shown that for the most part they belong to two families: atrioventricular septal defects (AVSD) and conotruncal cardiopathies (CTC). In these pathologies, the cardiopathies are almost always linked to other markers essential when performing morphological US examinations.

- Complex cardiopathies (those that will become critical at birth). In these cardiopathies, which are well tolerated in utero due to the presence of physiologic shunts, the karyotype and morphological studies are normal. After a very attentive verification of their isolated character during the morphological examination, the fetus is referred to the pediatric cardiologist. The pediatric cardiologist will then further clarify the diagnosis, considering the prognosis and organizing appropriate care at birth. In this category of critical cardiopathies we find complete transposition of the great vessels (TGV); this should be an obsession of every US specialist during examination of the fetus.

In this category of cardiopathies, you must equally eliminate the possibility of:

- an interruption of the aortic arch (IAA)
- an abnormal total anomalous pulmonary venous return (TAPVR).

When faced with certain cardiopathies whose prognosis is very bleak, or when the cardiopathy itself is a warning sign of a more complex pathology, the pediatric cardiologist might be led to propose a medical termination of pregnancy (MTP). Fetal pathologic verification is therefore highly recommended.[5] With the family's agreement, the fetal pathologist searches for those markers that were not visible during US in order to determine if the cardiopathy can be classified as a genetic syndrome or association. The results of this research allow us to propose appropriate genetic counseling for future pregnancies.

> Half of the observed cardiopathies, with a frequency which has been consistently estimated at around 8 per 1000 births,[6,7] will only develop after hemodynamic modifications take place after birth. Only 1 fetus in 250 carries a cardiopathy that is possibly detectable in utero.

Recently, systematic US investigations of nuchal translucency (NT) at a gestational age of 12 weeks improved our prognostic abilities. After a raised NT value has been observed in the chromosomally normal fetus, the frequency of congenital heart disease (CHD) in these types of fetuses is also increased.[8,9] Just as in women who have a high risk of cardiopathy,[10] this can justify a fetal control around 18 gestational weeks or earlier[11] necessitating further examinations, especially in those countries where legislation does not allow an MTP except at its earliest stages.

In pregnancies without particular problems, the heart is systematically verified by morphological US at 22 weeks. Even when considered normal at this stage, the heart should be observed by growth US at 32 weeks. It seems clear that a strictly architectural pathology could not have begun to form between the 22nd and 32nd gestational weeks. For instance, a heart found to have an AVSD at a gestational age of 32 weeks was not normal earlier at 22 weeks; AVSD was present during the very first weeks of development. On the other hand, certain pathologies, even architectural ones, evolve in relation to flow. Pathologies such as these, which were invisible or poorly visualized, even passing unseen at 22 gestational weeks, can be individually observed at 32 weeks.

The result of such screening on the detection of CHD has been studied in Europe,[12] showing variations depending on the different methods and protocols in use. The countries having the best results are those where every woman has access to three US examinations (at 12 weeks for NT, around the 22nd week with a morphological examination, and the third examination at 32 gestational weeks to check growth and re-verify the morphology). In certain countries, where legislation has modified this practice, some centers have developed new incidences[13] (such as the three-vessel view) or have perfected new techniques (3D and 4D).[14] Although the routine application of these new methods remains limited, for the moment, once the technical difficulties have been overcome they will provide us with a solid basis for our knowledge.

Though rarely seen the predictive value of cardiac anomalies is an extremely important warning sign of other anomalies (when considering all CHD taken together, and in relation to the increased risk of chromosomal abnormalities). Because of these observations, when a cardiopathy is discovered using US, the practice of determining the karyotype becomes indispensable.[15] This is especially true because we now know that there are chromosomal anomalies in more than 33% of the cases studied (more than 15% in those cases where the cardiopathy appears isolated, and around 40% in those cases reported when the morphological examination reveals an associated anomaly).[16]

A complementary examination researching the deletion of chromosome 22q11 will be requested in the case of conotruncal malformations.[17] Here we see the important role the fetal pathologic examination plays when a pregnancy has been medically terminated for an "isolated" cardiopathy. Markers that were difficult or impossible to see during US can be present here, such as a dysmorphology or visceral situs anomalies. This will allow us to identify known or unknown polymalformation syndromes.

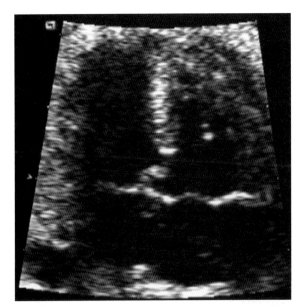

Figure 1.1   Apical four-chamber view. Complete AVSD associating an ASD ostium primum with LIAVV and inlet VSD.

The frequency of karyotype anomalies also varies depending on the type of cardiopathy observed. We know that there is an occurrence of nearly 40% of trisomy 21 (T21) when an AVSD has been diagnosed.[18] For instance, when faced with complete AVSD (Figs 1.1 and 1.2), if the karyotype is not known, we should first verify fetal nasal bone (FNB).[19,20] It is important to note that an incorrect size or absence (Fig. 1.3) here, like an amesophalangy or a brachymesophalangy (Fig. 1.4), represents an important complementary element. It is equally important to remember that in cases of

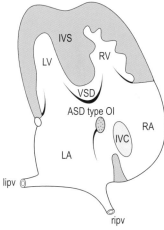

Figure 1.2   Illustration of the same complete AVSD as in Figure 1.1 (apical view).

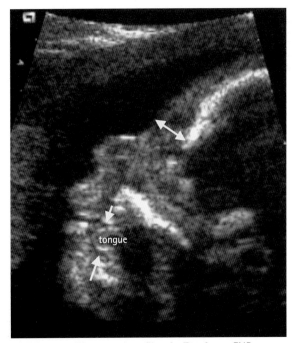

Figure 1.3   Ultrasound profile of a T21 fetus; FNB absent. Note the lingual protrusion and the width of the prefrontal panicle (arrows).

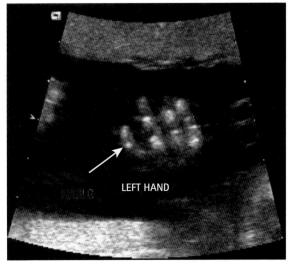

Figure 1.4   Echogram of the hand of a T21 fetus with a brachymesophalangy (arrow) of the fifth digit.

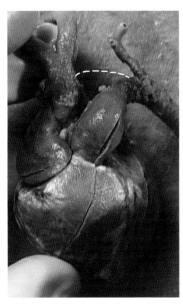

Figure 1.5   Heart with a B2 IAA (dotted line) in a fetus with 22q11 deletion.

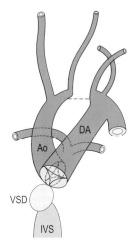

Figure 1.6   Diagram of an IAA in a B2 fetus.

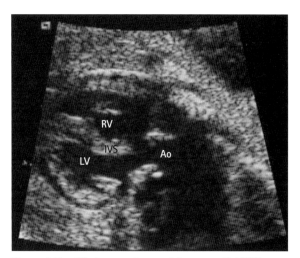

Figure 1.7   US view: aorta overriding an outlet VSD.

interruption of the aortic arch (IAA) and coarctation of the B2 type (Figs 1.5 and 1.6),[21] which is a rare form of CTC, over 80% show a microdeletion in 22q11. Note also that in this particular CTC, provoked by a neural crest pathology,[22] the presence of an outlet VSD is *constant* (Fig. 1.7).

Attention given to these confirmed anatomic findings in fetal pathology allow us to be sensitive to the presence of these pathologies, guiding our investigations. We know that:

- In all forms of AVSD, true linearity of the atrioventricular valves (AVV) is always found with a consistent absence of offsetting.[23]
- In all CTCs there exists a constant outlet VSD caused in most cases by misalignment, with the subsequent loss of left ventricle–aorta (LV–Ao) alignment.

These findings have led us to focus our research, not on *all* the important pathologic elements that *could be* detected, but rather to identify the *minimum diagnostic criteria necessary*, which, when used through systematic US examination of the heart, allow us eliminate these suspect pathologies.

The key to understanding our methodology is that it is based on the verification of *the* criteria for normality allowing us to eliminate any suspicion of important pathologies, rather than a strict sequential, segmental analysis,[24] which creates an exhaustive search for each marker or each sign of any individual pathology. To use our method, we must clearly identify those elements that allow this verification, determining which views and images make this possible.

Criteria for normality

1. In the four-chamber view (Fig. 1.8), the crux of the heart, with the two normally offset auricular–ventricular septal leaflets, allows us to eliminate the presence of the AVC,[25] which is a well-known marker for T21, as well as other pathologies.
2. One or two pulmonary veins extending into the left atrium (LA) in the four-chamber view rules out the eventuality of TAPVR.[26]

3. A septal–aortic alignment in several incidences used to explore outflow allows us to rule out the diagnosis of VSD by misalignment, a type of VSD present in a large majority of CTCs (Fig. 1.9).

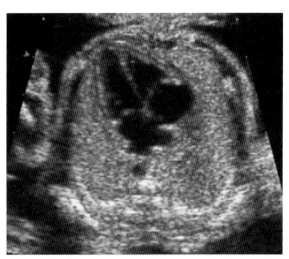

Figure 1.8 On this view of four normal chambers we see normal offsetting and visualization of two pulmonary veins. We do not find any form of the AVSD spectrum or TAPVR.

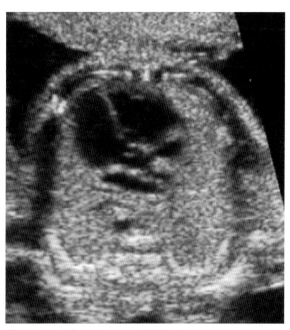

Figure 1.9 On this normal LV–Ao view we see a normal septal aortic continuity. There is no VSD by misalignment nor any atrioventricular discordance.

4. Two concordant and crossed arched vessels viewed together statically (Fig. 1.10), and one after the other in dynamic views, should allow us to eliminate the diagnosis of TGV.[27]

5. A complete arch of regular diameter with normal branching, seen eventually in color Doppler (Fig. 1.11), rules out the suspicion of IAA. Its origin, at the center of the heart, is a negative argument to eliminate the diagnosis of TGV. Size here reassures us of the balance between the aorta and pulmonary trunk (PT), due to the fact that this is usually modified in most instances of CTC as well as right- or left-tract hypoplasias.

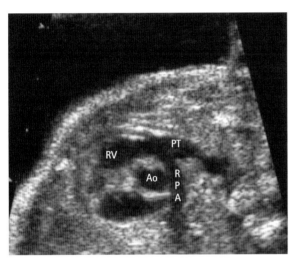

Figure 1.10   In this US view there is a normal ventricular–arterial concordance. There is no TGV or ventricular–arterial discordance.

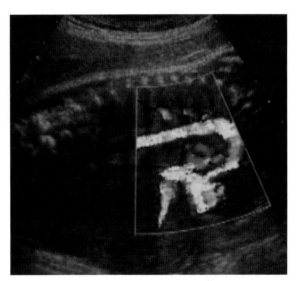

Figure 1.11   In this US view the aorta is seen rising in the center of the heart with a regular arch. IAA; TGV, and CTC are unlikely.

!!! ATTENTION !!!

The ultrasound specialist who detects a cardiac anomaly during morphological ultrasound investigations, rather than attempting a precise cardiopathologic diagnosis, should continue the examination by searching for *associated signs* through a thorough and well-directed morphological examination.

REVIEW

Several points concerning the development, anatomy, and hemodynamic qualities of the fetal heart will improve our understanding and make the examination easier.

Development

The heart—whose architecture is definitive at a gestational age of 10 weeks in a fetus with a cranial rump length (CRL) of less than 4 cm—is the size of a grain of rice and beats at more than 160 per minute.

Its evolution is influenced by developmental and lateralization genes, neural crests, and the flow which begins to pass through it by the fifth week of gestation.

Seeing this in a schematic way, the initial tube develops out of the islands of angioforming cells whose origin is splanchnopleuric and which are situated on the anterior pole of the embryo. Next, during the phase of delimitation, the explosive growth of the cephalic pole induces a coiling of the anterior pole of the embryo, causing the cardiac primordium to pivot by 180°. This then becomes ventral in relation to the cephalic pole and the stomodeum (the future mouth). The most anterior part of these tubes, formed by a symmetric tube pair which has become fused at their most distal section in the pericardiac cavity, becomes the cardiac tube itself. This tube then binds to the venous cardinal and vitellin systems (Fig. 1.12).

The intrapericardiac portion of the fused tube, due to its growth in a limited space, will normally form a right loop (Fig. 1.13).[28] This will then

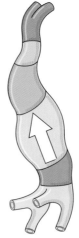
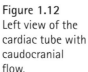
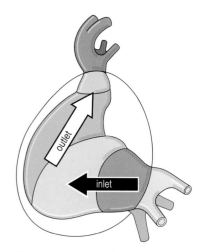

Figure 1.12 Left view of the cardiac tube with caudocranial flow.

Figure 1.13   Left view of the tube after the formation of the right loop showing inlet and outlet flows.

develop into an organ that is both uneven and asymmetric.

The initial section, situated before the loop or inlet, is formed by a primitive atrium receiving the venous returns and communicating through a unique anulus, called the atrioventricular canal (AVC), with the primitive ventricle.

The distal section, situated after the loop, or outlet, is followed by the arterial system which is formed out of the common arterial trunk (CAT) and then followed by the aortic arches.

The evolution of this tube, with its chambers connected in series, is made by the compartmentalization of the inlet section. This section is located before the loop in a relatively orthogonal way in four chambers with:

- Auricular septation with two septa. The septum primum will only close at the end of AVC development. The initial AVC will produce two offset anuli (Figs 1.14 and 1.15).
- At the same time the closing of the inlet section of the interventricular septum (IVS) will take place.

These phenomena, which are far more complex in reality, are still the focus of much fundamental research.[29]

We now arrive at the formation of parallel inlet tracts (Fig. 1.16), situated in the same plane.

It is this inlet plane that we have selected as the "optimal" four-chamber US view.

The outlet section undergoes far more complex modifications. Located after the loop, the distal section of the tube in which outflow is seen, is under the influence of neural crests.[30] Here:

- The closing of the interventricular septum's outflow section occurs, which is located under the CAT. It appears more complex than the closing of the inflow septum (Fig. 1.17). This septum, with alignment, closes under the aorta, while the conal or infundibular septum separates the two great vessels.
- Above the outlet septum, the walling in and spiraling of the common arterial trunk develops

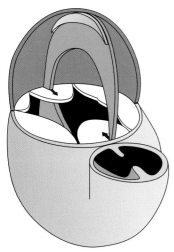

Figure 1.14   Anterior view: vertical diagram of the heart before the division of the AVC and the initial CAT.

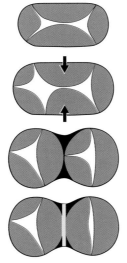

Figure 1.15   Anterior left view with a diagram of the stages of the transformation of the AVC into two annuli.

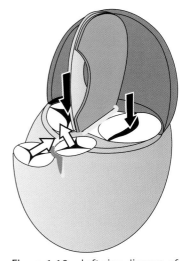

Figure 1.16   Left view diagram of the "verticalized" heart: septation achieved. Black parallel arrows represent the inlet flow; the orthogonal white arrows represent the outlet flow.

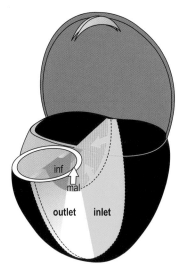

Figure 1.17 Diagram of the "verticalized" and opened heart. Localization of the inlet septum (yellow) and the outlet septum (alignment septum in white; infundibular in purple).

into two crossed vessels (Figs 1.18–1.23) They develop like this, above the alignment septum, each one out of its own outflow tract. These two crossed and arched vessels are separated by the infundibular or conal septum. Initially, in continuity with the right outlet flow, the aorta should be joined eventually to the left chamber to ensure left outlet flow.

The vessels have orifices which are conjoined but orthogonal, situated in superimposed levels (Fig. 1.24). They are linked to vessels derived from the aortic arches. This 6° arch gives rise to the right outlet: the PT; the pulmonary arteries and ductus arteriosus (DA). The 4° arch gives rise to the left outlet: the aorta and right subclavian artery (Fig. 1.25).

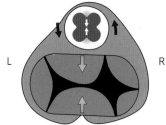

Figure 1.18 Posterior right view of the fetal heart after ablation of the atria and the great vessels, showing the initial CAT and initial AVC.

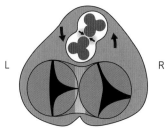

Figure 1.19 Intermediary stage. Evolution: partial AVC dominated by two vessels in the process of spiraling and wall development.

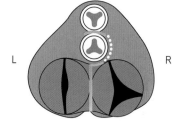

Figure 1.20 Final stage. Inlet: two anuli on the same plane; outlet: two conjoined, superimposed, and orthogonal anuli (the inlet septum is yellow, the membranous septum is green, the alignment septum is represented by a dotted line, and the infundibular is purple).

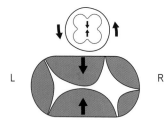

Figure 1.21 Diagram of Figure 1.18 as seen from the posterior right.

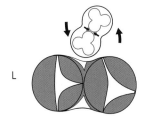

Figure 1.22 Diagram of Figure 1.19 as seen from the posterior right.

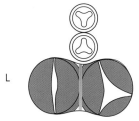

Figure 1.23 Diagram of Figure 1.20 as seen from the posterior right.

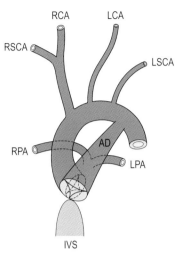

Figure 1.24   Diagram of the outlet vessels with conjoined and orthogonal annuli over a closed IVS.

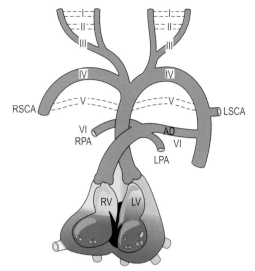

Figure 1.25   Evolution of the aortic arches: the 4° left arch becomes the aorta and the 6° arch becomes the pulmonary vessels (PT, PAs, and DA).

The position of the outlet tracts, with their superimposed orifices, initially has quasi-perpendicular trajectories whose objective is to join together the *same* vessel. This explains the necessity for multiple views using both static and dynamic methods in order to explore their subsequent trajectory.

By our understanding of these simple observations a verification of cardiac architecture involving several steps and at different levels can be performed: verification of position and that of the inlet and the outlet. These different steps become our guiding light, which, leading us from the normal to the pathologic, allows the development of a system for the classification of cardiopathies which is especially applicable in prenatal US examinations.

Anatomic ultrasound correlations

The heart—whose architecture is definitive by the time of its observation by US—has a size that varies between that of a chickpea (at 12 weeks) to that of an olive (at 22 weeks); by 32 weeks it is the size of an almond (Fig. 1.26).

Establishing the anatomic relationships within such a small organ is important, especially an organ

that beats between 120 and 160 times per minute. It is also important to recognize that these relationships within the fetal heart differ in certain points from those in the adult heart. During its fetal existence, the heart has a left axis which makes an angle of 45° with the anteroposterior axis.

> The heart is seen to be lying horizontally on the diaphragm, which is situated on the axial plane of the fetus.

This distinctive quality in relation to postnatal anatomy is explained by the volume of the fetal liver, and pulmonary vacuity (Fig. 1.27). The fetal heart is situated flat on the diaphragm, the apex directed to the left.

Apart from the positioning of the heart itself, it is essential to differentiate the inlet and outlet. (Figs 1.28–1.30).

The inlet involves the pulmonary venous return (PVR) (Fig. 1.31) and the systemic venous return (SVR), which enter respectively into the left atrium (LA) and right atrium (RA).

The primary element involved in the anchoring of the heart (the LA) is in a median position just before the spine. It is attached to the lungs (Figs 1.32 and 1.33) by the four pulmonary veins, which constitute

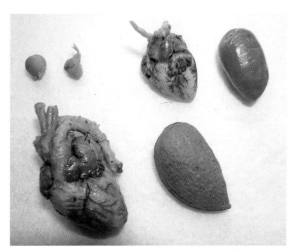

Figure 1.26 Comparison of the size of a fetal heart at 12, 22, and 32 weeks' gestation.

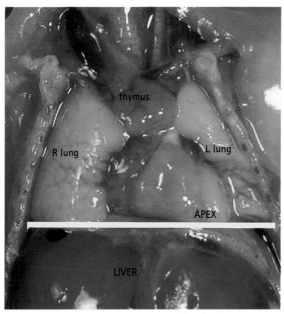

Figure 1.27 Fetal heart–lung block (HLB). The fetal heart is placed flat on the diaphragm (white line) with the apex pointed to the left.

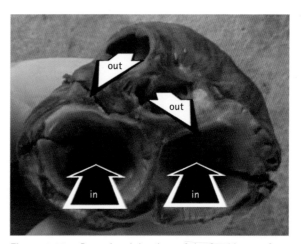

Figure 1.28 Posterior right view of the fetal heart after an ablation of the atria and the great vessels: inlet (black parallel arrows situated in the same plane); outlet (white orthogonal arrows seen in superimposed planes).

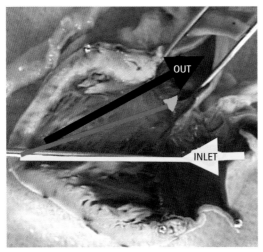

Figure 1.29   View of the fetal heart opened to the left: left inlet (yellow arrow) and outlet (black arrow). The red line, which rejoins the green triangle (representing the membranous septum), marks the limit between inlet and outlet.

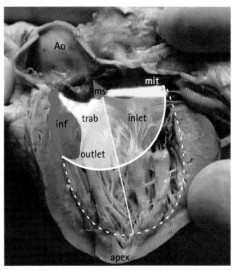

Figure 1.30   The same view as in Figure 1.29 on a "verticalized" heart opened to the left (inlet: yellow; outlet: trabecular in white; and infundibular or conal in purple).

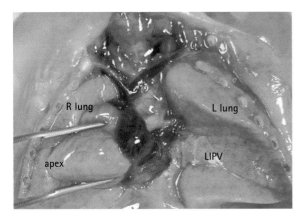

Figure 1.31   Heart–lung block, front view. Heart swung to the right, "exposing" the left inferior pulmonary vein.

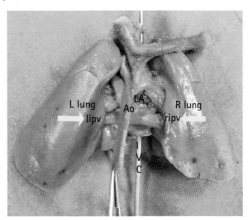

Figure 1.32   Heart–lung block, posterior view. Systemic venous return by the ICV and SCV as obtained by probe and the PVR as shown by the yellow arrows.

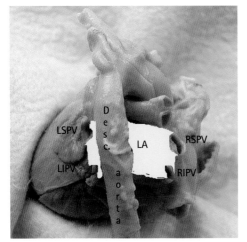

Figure 1.33   Fetal heart, posterior view. Left atrium in front of the descending aorta; venous return by the four pulmonary veins.

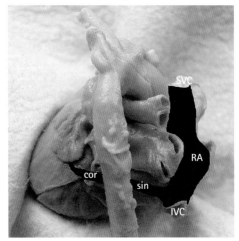

Figure 1.34   Fetal heart, posterior view. Systemic venous return into the RA by the SVC and IVC *and* the CS.

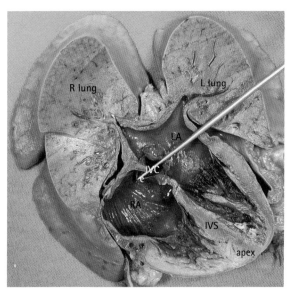

Figure 1.35   Heart–lung block cut at the level of the optimal four-chamber view (the apex and two inferior PVs). The probe shows the trajectory of oxygenated flow from the IVC towards the RA through the FO. e, eustachian valve.

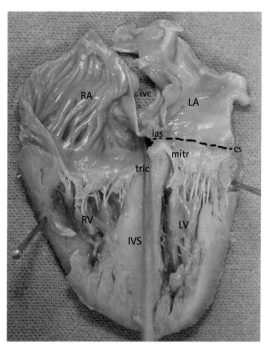

Figure 1.36   "Optimal" anatomic four-chamber view. The probe is here at the emergence of the CS in the RA. The dotted line marks the posterior trajectory of the CS in the left inter-atrioventricular groove.

the pulmonary venous return. The RA is right lateral, more anterior, and receives the systemic venous return. It is composed of three elements: the venae cavae, superior and inferior, which are situated in the cranial–caudal axis; and the coronary sinus (Fig. 1.34). This coronary sinus, which forms the SVR of the heart, heads towards the RA in the left atrioventricular groove.

Each inlet ventricular chamber should be in concordance with its homologous atrium: the RA with its right ventricular inflow chamber, and the same for the LA, which should be in concordance with the left ventricular inlet chamber. These four chambers, the two atrial and two ventricular inlet chambers, can be examined using the four-chamber view.

The "optimal" four-chamber view (Fig. 1.35)[25] is defined to give us a reference view for examining all the key points concerning inlet, at the same time creating reproducible observations that can be referred to later, and clearly understood both in terms of fetal pathology and US. Situated on the axial plane of the fetus, the view is defined by three reference points; these are the apex and the two inferior pulmonary veins.

On this "optimal" view we can verify that:

- The apex of the heart is formed by the left ventricle (LV), itself characterized by the smoothness of the septum in this cavity.
- The anterior right ventricle (RV), which is retrosternal, is characterized by its coarse trabeculations.
- The crux of the heart is where the septal leaflets of the AVVs can be seen inserted in an offset fashion. The tricuspid detaches from the IVS closer to the apex, and the leaflet is linked to this septum by a septal attachment. The septal leaflet of the mitral valve has no such septal attachment.

Note the situation of the coronary sinus (Fig. 1.36), which is cut at the level of its initial section in the atrioventricular groove between the LV and the RA. Arriving after a posterior trajectory in the groove entering the RA, it is in proximity to the base of the interatrial septum (IAS).

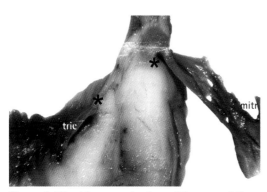

Figure 1.37   Macroscopic view of the crux of the heart: mitral leaflet without septal attachment whereas the tricuspid septal leaflet is "stuck" to the IVS in its initial section. The asterisks (*) mark the offset of the AV valves.

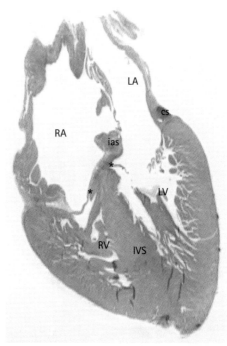

Figure 1.38   Histologic four-chamber view: Note the offsetting "*" in the insertion of the atrioventricular valves in the IVS.

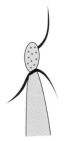

Figure 1.39 Diagram of the crux of the heart. The dotted line marks the portion of the IAS that is hyperechogenic because of the transversal section of fibers of the septum intermedium.

The crux of the heart

It is here we find the essential foundation for our key point used in screening for AVSD pathologies (Fig. 1.37). Using the histologic examination (Fig. 1.38) and its various components will allow us to understand the differences in echogenicity that are important in order to be able to interpret this correctly.[25]

- The anterior section of the IAS (the septum intermedium), where the valve of the foramen ovale (FO) is attached, is composed of muscular fibers that are transversally cut. It is thus echogenic no matter what US access is employed; it appears as a dotted image in this figure (Fig. 1.39).
- The fibers of the IVS are longitudinal to the axis of the septum; they are thus difficult to see by an apical incidence. When the ultrasonic beams are parallel, you can imagine observing a defect, whereas transverse access highlights this composition particularly well.
- The mitral leaflet, which is without attachment to the IVS, is of a fibrous nature and, in reality, is continuous with the septal tricuspid leaflet, which is of the same nature. Between the IAS and the IVS the septal portions of the two leaflets are linked by an oblique intermediary zone (see Fig. 1.36).[25]

Given its fibrous nature this zone should be seen in US as an oblique line, which, by the mirroring effect, appears hyperechogenic when it is approached perpendicularly. It will not be seen if the approach is made along its axis. **It is the obliqueness of the intermediate zone that is responsible for the impression of offsetting the valves.**

These specific histologic characteristics explain the constant echogenic character of the IAS ("the head" of the crux) and the poor visualization of the IVS apically.

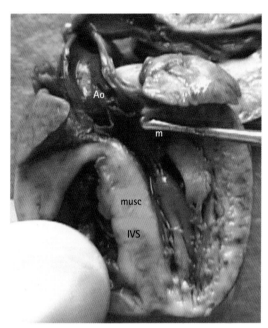

Figure 1.40 Macroscopic anatomic view of the apical long axis of the LV–Ao.

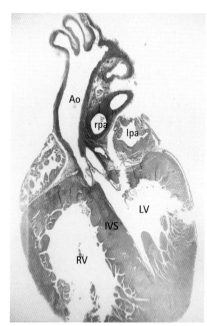

Figure 1.41 Histologic view of the apical incidence LV–Ao. Note the offsetting at the level of the septal–aortic musculofibrous continuity. The difference in constitution and size—the thick, muscular IVS and the thin, fibrous aortic wall—explains the "misalignment" that is already present, in the absence of the defect and which always occurs in the presence of a subaortic defect.

Outflow

This is composed of two arched tracts.

1. The left outlet uses the aorta (Figs 1.40 and 1.41), which begins in the center of the heart in continuity with the IVS, and also with the mitral anulus *and* the tricuspid anulus. The septal aortic continuity as well as the mitral aortic continuity are visible by a view which is close to the four-chamber view making an acute angle to them. The adjacency of the aortic and pulmonary anuli (conjoined but orthogonal) allows us to examine the two at once in the sagittal plane of the fetus by cutting the aortic anulus transversally and the pulmonary anulus longitudinally (Figs 1.42 and 1.43). This is the DA view.
2. The right outlet (Fig. 1.44) is brought about by the PT at the top of the infundibulum. It is thick and filled with muscular fibers, marking the clear discontinuity between the tricuspid anulus and the PT. The angle between the four-chamber view and the right outlet is clearly less acute than that made by the left inlet with the left outlet due to the interposition of the infundibulum.

The great vessels

The aorta and PT arise out of the superimposed rings in an orthogonal direction. They will join together on the same vessel (Fig. 1.45), the descending aorta which runs in front and to the left of the spine.

The arches

The aortic arch, beginning in the center of the heart, is described as an arch formed by an acute angle. The ductal arch takes a trajectory that is practically rectilinear, anteroposterior, beginning in the retrosternal region with a ductal arch of an obtuse angle. Soon after its emergence from the RV, the PT gives rise, on its posterior side, to the two pulmonary arteries (PA); the right PA wraps the aortic root. After branching, the PT becomes the DA sharing a short, almost parallel, trajectory which can be best seen with the three-vessel view

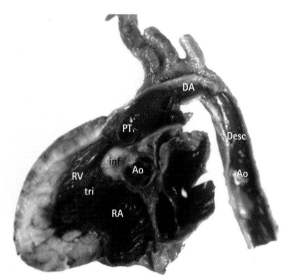

Figure 1.42   Anatomic view—the "arterial duct view" (AD)—where the aorta is cut transversally and the PT longitudinally.

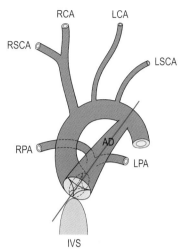

Figure 1.43   Situation of the viewing plane in the AD view (green line) on a diagram of the great vessels.

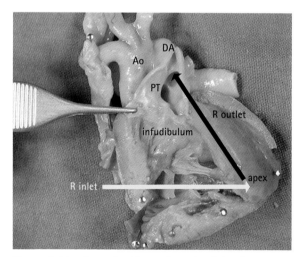

Figure 1.44   Open fetal heart from the right: departure of the PT above the infundibulum. This is why the angle between the right inlet and right outlet is less acute than that between the left inlet and left outlet.

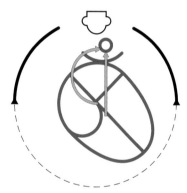

Figure 1.45   Diagram of the fetal heart with the US reference points (complete ribs, apex and two pulmonary veins, and the aorta). The arrows represent the great vessels leaving at the same level to rejoin the aorta by different trajectories.

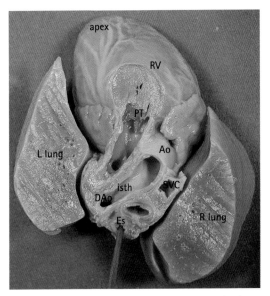

Figure 1.46 Superior view of the HLB anatomic view at the level of the three vessels. The pulmonary trunk and aorta are cut longitudinally, and the SVC is cut transversally.

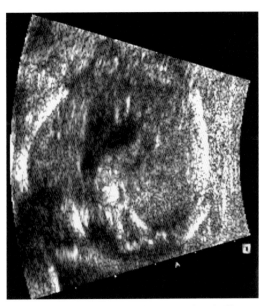

Figure 1.47 Corresponding US view to that in Figure 1.46. The three-vessels view or the view of the arches.

(Figs 1.46 and 1.47). This view—axial and slightly oblique—longitudinally cuts the upper part of the arches and transversally the right superior vena cava (SVC). From right to left we can see the SVC, the aorta and the DA.

The junction of the great vessels with the descending aorta explains why they can both be observed through a left paravertebral window, giving us the possibility of a posterior approach through the three-vessel view as we have for the aortic arch.

The exploration of the great vessels, combined like a *guédoufle* (Fig. 1.48), can be visualized dynamically by passing from one tract to the other (Fig. 1.49). Depending on the angle, whether it is apical or oblique (Figs 1.50 and 1.51), the anatomic aspects of the views differ.

If the complete verification of the two great vessels, both statically and dynamically, is not possible, the certainty of a normal ventricular arterial concordance is reassuring. When we see RV–PT or LV–Ao concordance, it allows us to assume, by definition, that transposition of the great vessels has not occurred – the ventriculo-arterial discordance being the hallmark of this pathology.

In fact, an RV–PT concordance (Figs 1.52 and 1.53) is always accompanied by an LV–Ao concordance because while two appendages of the same type in isomerisms can exist, when there are two ventricles they are always different.

> Knowledge of anatomic relationships allows us to understand that, contrary to the inlet tract with its four chambers situated in the same axial plane allowing exploration by the four-chamber view alone, the verification of the outlet, with its crossed and superimposed vessels, needs—more often than not—*varied and complementary views,* which are both static and dynamic.

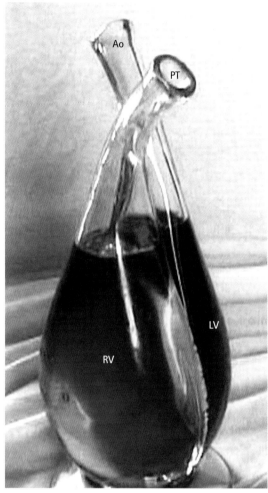

Figure 1.48   *Guédoufle*: the side containing oil represents the right outflow tract (RV–PT), the side containing vinegar represents the left outflow tract (LV–Ao).

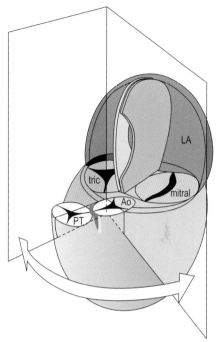

Figure 1.49   Diagram of the "verticalized" heart showing sweeping movements of the RV–PT/LV–Ao.

Several fetal hemodynamic elements

Fetal blood flow begins early, being identifiable by the fifth gestational week. This flow is an important element in the modeling of the heart. First linear, and then caudal–cranial, the flow undergoes an angulation during the formation of the heart loop which allows us to differentiate it in Figure 1.54: an inlet flow directed anteriorly and towards the left, in an axial plane, parallel to the diaphragm and in a continuum followed by an outlet flow located after the right loop and in a more cranial direction.

While the architecture is definite by 10 weeks, the hemodynamics develop throughout pregnancy,[31] resulting in the architecture of certain pathologies. The two physiologic shunts should be noted. The particularity of the fetal–maternal circulation rests on the existence of these shunts which close soon after birth. They are:

- The shunt passing through the FO from the RA (Fig. 1.55) towards the LA is a caudal–cranial flow.
- The shunt passing through the DA from the PT towards the descending aorta is an antero-posterior flow.

Two simple concepts help us to understand this:
1. The fetal heart ejects the flow it receives.
2. The size of the chamber or vessel is proportional to the flow that crosses it.

Normally, one sees the convergence of the systemic venal return (SVR) at the level of the entrance of the inlet tract in the RA. This includes:

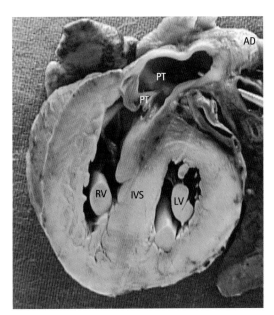

Figure 1.50   *Guédoufle*: view of the ventricles with right outflow, RV–PT. Notice the moderator band in the right ventricle and two papillary muscles; one inferior, the other superior in the left ventricle.

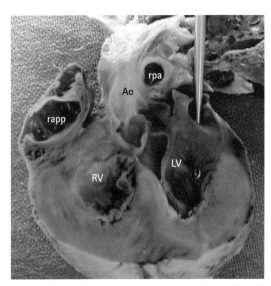

Figure 1.51   *Guédoufle*: view of ventricles with left outflow: LV–Ao. The right pulmonary artery is cut transversally while wrapping the aortic root. The probe is in the left appendage.

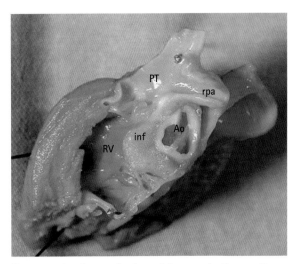

Figure 1.52   Anatomic view of the vessels, the small axis. The RPA is cut longitudinally while wrapping the aortic root. There is a ventricular arterial concordance.

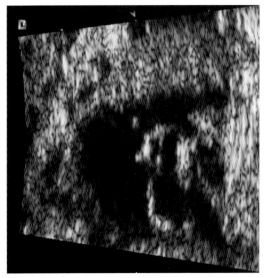

Figure 1.53   Ultrasound view of the same short axis view as in Figure 1.52.

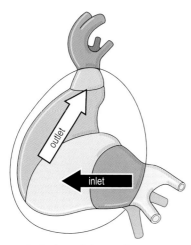

Figure 1.54   Left view of the cardiac tube after the right loop: identification of the inlet and outlet.

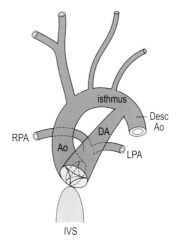

Figure 1.56   Diagram of fetal hemodynamics: the ductus arteriosus.

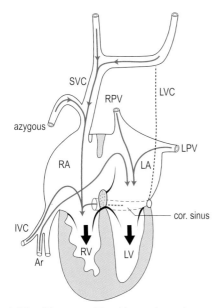

Figure 1.55   Diagram of fetal hemodynamics: venous return and inlet. The red line shows the oxygenated flow coming from the IVC towards the left tract through the FO. Ar-Arantius canal.

- The flow of the SVC draining the upper part of the body.
- The majority of the flow of the inferior vena cava (IVC) draining the lower half.
- The coronary sinus (CS), which is the venous return of the heart.

The PVR converges into the LA by the four pulmonary veins, but also the oxygenated flow of the IVC. The oxygenated flow arrives by the umbilical vein and is then, in part, shunted towards the liver through the canal of Arantius. Here it reaches the LA where it is directed by the Eustachian valve through the FO; this is the first physiologic shunt.

The balance of the RA/LA shunt is manifested by the normal presence of the valve of the FO in the LA, pushed by the flow.

The inlet flow then enters the chambers of the RV and LV, respectively, entering through the tricuspid and mitral valves.

Examples of inlet pathologies

Several examples of pathologies at the level of the inflow tract include:

- The lack of balance between the atria caused by an excess of inlet flow in the RA. For example:
  - In the case of a partially abnormal PVR into a persistent left SVC, the coronary sinus (CS) drains a part of the pulmonary flow towards the RA. In certain circumstances the CS can be dilated to the point where it obstructs the entry flow into the LV.[32]
  - In the case of tricuspid atresia, due to the failure of inflow entering the RV, the increase in right flow "pushes" the valve of the FO, which being "forced," appears to be even more deviated to the left than normal.

- Inversion of the RA/LA flow in case of obstacles in the left tracts, an example being mitral atresia where there is an inversion of interauricular flow, the valve of the FO being in the RA instead of the LA.

A lack of balance between the atriums has repercussions on the ventricles.

> Inlet anomalies are found using the four-chamber view.

Normally the outlets develop out of the two balanced ventricles separated by an intact septum and composed of two crossed vessels of comparable diameter, though the diameter of the PT is slightly superior to that of the aorta. These crossed vessels are superimposed with their conjoined anuli situated in two orthogonal planes (Fig. 1.56). Despite their different points of origin, the great vessels rejoin the same vessel, the descending aorta, situated in the back of the left section of the LA. The PT, after the emergence of the two pulmonary arteries (the RPA and LPA), is called the arterial duct; this is the second shunt. It has a rectilinear transit, anteroposterior, until reaching the descending aorta. The aorta describes a large, hook-shaped curve—the arch—before joining the descending aorta.

Flow in these two arches should occur in the *same* direction, and any inversion of flow in either of these vessels is pathologic.[33]

Examples of outlet pathologies

When one of the two outlet tracts is stenotic or atresic, the other is dilated.

> A large aorta is always accompanied by a small PA (and vice versa).

For the above reason, during the Doppler examination on the three-vessel view, we sometimes find the direction of the flow reversed in the ducts, which signifies a *reverse flow* of one of these vessels coming from the other; **this is something that is always pathologic**.

If the ventricles situated under the unbalanced great vessels are balanced, we can equally assume the existence of a VSD, for example a large aorta coming out of the two ventricles, seen as being balanced in the four-chamber view, is inevitably overriding a VSD. It should be noted that in the case of an overriding aorta, the axis of the inlet of the heart is modified (with an axis steeper than 45°).[34]

> These outlet anomalies can be researched using all views that explore outlet flow.

One should especially take note of aortic physiology. The coronary vessels, which are indispensable for support of the cardiac muscle, must at least receive minimal flow. In the case of aortic atresia, a retrograde vascularization by the DA is indispensable.

During the fetal period, this retrograde vascularization permits a tolerance for a cardiopathy called "duct dependent" until the closing of the DA after birth.

Other cardiopathies are also duct dependent, that is to say, dependent on the maintenance of a permeability of the CA. Their prognosis[34] depends on the quality of care the newborn receives in appropriate settings. This is the case for TGV[35] and certain cases of pulmonary atresia with VSD (PA with OS). In the case of TGV, the perinatal hemodynamic problems involving the DA and the FO require a follow-up with intensive cardiopediatric care. At the same time, in certain forms of PA with OS the initial portion of the PT is either difficult to observe or nonexistent, and the pulmonary vascularization is accomplished by collateral aortic arteries or main aortic–pulmonary collateral arteries (MAPCA).[36] This systemic palliative vascularization can continue after birth, but its long-term consequences are harmful.

APPLICATION TO FETAL CARDIOPATHIES

Out of this very simplified vision of fetal development, anatomy, and hemodynamics, we created a classification that is of practical use in the investigation of the fetal heart.

This practical classification of prenatal screening begins with three principal categories:

- position anomalies
- inlet anomalies
- outlet anomalies.

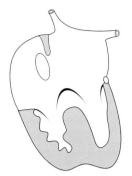

Figure 1.57   Diagram of the major form of complete AVSD: very incomplete auricular septation with a large septal defect.

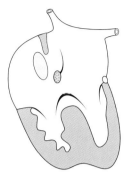

Figure 1.58   Diagram of complete AVSD with intermedium septum (round and pointed with the departure of the flap valve).

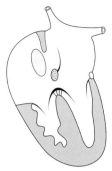

Figure 1.59   Diagram of complete AVSD with attachment of the bridging leaflets on the top of the ventricular crest.

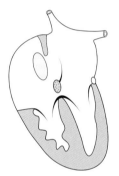

Figure 1.60   Diagram of partial AVSD: IAS defect (ostium primum type) associated with a mitral cleft.

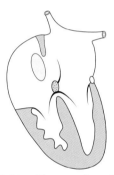

Figure 1.61   Diagram of partial AVSD: IVS defect.

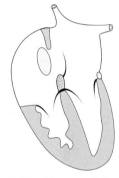

Figure 1.62   Diagram of the minor form AVSD: LIAVV without defect.

Certain complex cardiopathes belong to several of the above categories. In each of these categores further anomalies associated with flow can be a part of the cardiopathy, increasing the severity. Examples are described below.

The concept of the architectural spectrum

An important idea coming out of our observations of fetal pathology is the concept of a spectrum of malformations. Of course there is not *one* type of complete AVSD and *one* type of partial AVSD any more than there is *one* type of normal heart; instead there is a large spectrum of AVSD malformations, with numerous intermediary forms.

We begin with a complete form of AVSD with a total absence of closing of the initial AVSD. Here we see that the large defect (Fig. 1.57) is due to the confluence of the ASD ostium primum and of the inlet VSD above the atrioventricular bridging leaflet, which remains in common (Figs 1.58 and 1.59). The minor form, which we discovered and published earlier,[23,24] exhibits the absence of any offsetting between the AVV, with the linear insertion of these valves, or an LIAVV without any defect (Fig. 1.62). This also includes all other forms of partial AVSD; one type involves a mitral cleft associated with an ASD ostium primum (Fig. 1.60) or an inlet VSD (Fig. 1.61).

Building on the idea of these spectrum classifications we come to their practical application. We search systematically for warning signs which are the "lowest common denominator," or the slightest sign, of these pathologies. In the case of the AVSD spectrum it appears to be the absence of a normal offsetting of the septal valves at the level of

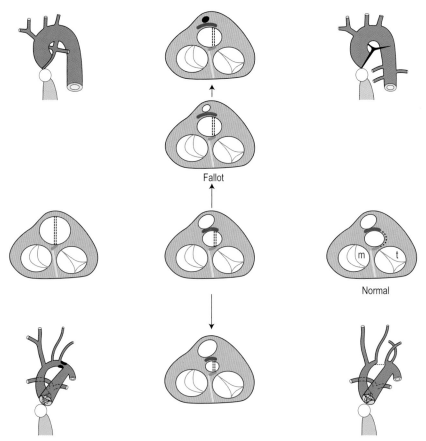

Figure 1.63   CTC spectrum shown starting with the major form (the CAT) to the minor form (the outlet septal defect). In the case of an anterior swing this is seen from tetralogy of Fallot to PA with OS. In the case of posterior swing, this is the syndrome of coarctation to IAA.

the crux of the heart, or linear insertion. This observation is more important, and easier to see, than the defects associated with AVSD itself.

> In all cardiopathies of the AVSD spectrum the AVV are linear.

For the CTC spectrum (Fig. 1.63), the outlet VSD is constant, usually by misalignment, with a loss of the septal–aortic continuity. This type of mis-alignment VSD is found in the great majority of anomalies of this spectrum including the CAT. There is also a spectrum which is defined by the direction of the swing of the infundibular septum. When there is an anterior swing that creates a progressive stenosis of the PT, we have a range of pathologies from tetralogy of Fallot (ToF) to PA with OS. In

the case of a posterior swing of the infundibular septum, where it is the aorta which experiences stenosis, we observe (at the mild end of the spectrum) a syndrome of aortic coarctation through to (on the severe end of this same spectrum) an IAA. Concerning a posterior swing, the VSD observed is more frequently infundibular, thus very difficult to detect by echo. **When we find ourselves in this situation, it is primarily the asymmetry of the vessel diameter that attracts our attention**.

Our concept of spectrums exists equally for the following types:

- A spectrum of recurring familial cardiopathies. In certain familial hypoplasia of the left tract the spectrum can even reach extreme forms of LV hypoplasia (mitral atresia associated with or without aortic atresia) as well as simple bicuspid aorta, often ignored or asymptomatic, but which must be considered as a minor feature of the same disease.

- There is also a hemodynamic spectrum, which explains the evolutionary character of certain pathologies during the course of the pregnancy. An example is the evolution during pregnancy of a minor form of ToF into a major form such as PA with OS.

This system of classification does not rely on clinical knowledge, as do postnatal cardiology classifications, instead it is based on our extensive anatomic experience of fetal hearts. In effect, the cardiopathies of chromosomal anomalies, associations, sequences and polymalformation syndromes, which form the basis for decisions to medically interrupt pregnancy, for the most part, belong to the families of cardiopathies and major forms of the different spectrums listed above. They are very different from the pathologies seen by the pediatric cardiologist post-natally. To further underline and simplify this idea, we will now discuss several important points.

Certain simple anatomic warning signs are rarely used systematically, even though they optimize the examination itself.

Here are three examples:

- Two contiguous vessels of equal diameter, parallel at the abdominal level and behind the RA, signal an impairment of the anomalous SVR with interruption of the suprarenal portion of the IVC.[37] This sign, very evocative of a visceral–atrial heterotaxia (VAH) with a right isomerism, is much easier to detect than the complex associated cardiopathies which are frequent, but far more difficult to diagnose.
- A right descending aorta is much easier to see on the four-chamber view than on the three-vessel view,[38] and it is an excellent warning sign of CTC.
- The modification of the axis of the IVS,[34] used in fetal pathology to judge asymmetry when inspecting an anatomic specimen, is equally easy to observe in US when we actually look for it.

Etiologic orientation

Each family of cardiac pathologies is related to a type of fetal pathology and thus determines the morphological examination.

Faced with a position anomaly, we search for the normality of the karyotype[39] and look for other vascular and/or morphological elements which are frequent in VAH.

Faced with an inlet anomaly belonging to the spectrum of AVSD, we first search, before the karyotype is known, for signs associated with T21[18] and that of other chromosomal pathologies. If the karyotype is known to be normal,[40] we must rather consider VAH and other syndromes, especially skeletal ones.

Faced with an outlet VSD, of a conotruncal variety, after searching for markers associated with the number of the chromosomal abnormalities, we look for those associated with deletions of the chromosome 22q11,[17] then, if the results are negative, we search for signs of malformations.

We are not going to touch on rhythm or structural abnormalities at this time. These pathologies, which are very infrequent, modify the cardiac rhythm or the echogenicity of the heart. For this reason, they always attract attention, and should be referred immediately to the expertise of the pediatric cardiologist.

References

1. Yates RS. The influence of prenatal diagnosis on postnatal outcome in patients with structural congenital heart disease. Prenat Diagn 2004; 24(13):1143–1149.
2. Khoshnood B, De Vigan C, Vodovar V et al. Trends in prenatal diagnosis, pregnancy termination, and perinatal mortality of newborns with congenital heart disease in France, 1983–2000: a population-based evaluation. Pediatrics 2005; 115(1):95–101.
3. Sharland GK. Routine fetal cardiac screening: what are we doing and what shall we do? Prenat Diagn 2004; 24(13):1123–1129.
4. Tennstedt C, Hufnagl P, Korner H et al. Fetal autopsy: the most important contribution of pathology in a center for perinatal medicine. Fetal Diagn Ther 2001; 16(6):384–393.
5. Piercecchi-Marti MD, Liprandi A, Sigaudy S et al. Value of fetal autopsy after medical termination of pregnancy. Forensic Sci Int 2004; 144(1):7–10.
6. Mitchell SC, Korones SB, Berendes HW. Congenital heart disease in 56,109 births. Incidence and natural history. Circulation 1971; 43(3):323–332.
7. Avagliano L, Grillo C, Prioli MA. Congenital heart disease: a retrospective study of their frequency. Minerva Ginecol 2005; 57(2):171–178.

8. Bahado-Singh RO, Wapner R, Thom E et al. Elevated first-trimester nuchal translucency increases the risk of congenital heart defects. Am J Obstet Gynecol 2005; 192(5):1357–1361.

9. Souka AP, von Kaisenberg CS, Hyett JA et al. Increased nuchal translucency with normal karyotype. Am J Obstet Gynecol 2005; 192(4):1005–1021 (review). Erratum in: Am J Obstet Gynecol 2005; 192(6):2096.

10. Comas Gabriel C, Galindo A, Martinez JM et al. Early prenatal diagnosis of major cardiac anomalies in a high-risk population. Prenat Diagn 2002; 22(7):586–593.

11. Yagel S, Achiron R, Ron M et al. Transvaginal ultrasonography at early pregnancy cannot be used alone for targeted organ ultrasonographic examination in a high-risk population. Am J Obstet Gynecol 1995; 172(3):971–975.

12. Stoll C, Dott B, Alembik Y, De Geeter B. Evaluation and evolution during time of prenatal diagnosis of congenital heart diseases by routine fetal ultrasonographic examination. Ann Genet 2002; 45(1):21–27.

13. Yagel S, Arbel R, Anteby EY et al. The three vessels and trachea view (3VT) in fetal cardiac scanning. Ultrasound Obstet Gynecol 2002; 20(4):340–345.

14. Deng J, Rodeck CH. New fetal cardiac imaging techniques. Prenat Diagn 2004; 24(13):1092–1103.

15. Moore JW, Binder GA, Berry R. Prenatal diagnosis of aneuploidy and deletion 22q11.2 in fetuses with ultrasound detection of cardiac defects. Am J Obstet Gynecol 2004; 191(6):2068–2073.

16. Wimalasundera RC, Gardiner HM. Congenital heart disease and aneuploidy. Prenat Diagn 2004; 24(13):1116–1122.

17. Boudjemline Y, Fermont L, Le Bidois J et al. Prevalence of 22q11 deletion in fetuses with conotruncal cardiac defects: a 6-year prospective study. J Pediatr 2001; 138(4):520–524.

18. Langford K, Sharland G, Simpson J. Relative risk of abnormal karyotype in fetuses found to have an atrioventricular septal defect (AVSD) on fetal echocardiography. Prenat Diagn 2005; 25(2):137–139.

19. Cicero S, Sacchini C, Rembouskos G, Nicolaides KH. Sonographic markers of fetal aneuploidy: a review. Placenta 2003; 24(suppl B):S88–S98.

20. Viossat P, Cans C, Marchal-André D et al. Role of "subtle" ultrasonographic signs during antenatal screening for trisomy 21 during the second trimester of pregnancy: meta-analysis and CPDPN protocol of the Grenoble University Hospital. J Gynecol Obstet Biol Reprod (Paris) 2005; 34(3 Pt 1):215–231 (in French).

21. Volpe P, Marasini M, Caruso G et al. 22q11 deletions in fetuses with malformations of the outflow tracts or interruption of the aortic arch: impact of additional ultrasound signs. Prenat Diagn 2003; 23(9):752–757.

22. Kirby ML, Turnage KL 3rd, Hays BM. Characterization of conotruncal malformations following ablation of "cardiac" neural crest. Anat Rec 1985; 213(1):87–93.

23. Fredouille C, Piercecchi-Marti MD, Liprandi A et al. Linear insertion of atrioventricular valves without septal defect: a new anatomical landmark for Down's syndrome? Fetal Diagn Ther 2002; 17(3):188–192. Erratum in: Fetal Diagn Ther 2002; 17(5):292.

24. Carvalho JS. Ho SY. Shinebourne EA. Sequential segmental analysis in complex fetal cardiac abnormalities: a logical approach to diagnosis. Ultrasound Obstet Gynecol 2005; 26(2):105–111.

25. Fredouille C, Baschet N, Develay-Morice J-E et al. Linear insertion of the atrioventricular valves without defect. Arch Mal Coeur Vaiss 2005; 98(5):549–555 (in French).

26. Allan LD, Sharland GK. The echocardiographic diagnosis of totally anomalous pulmonary venous connection in the fetus. Heart 2001; 85(4):433–437.

27. De Geeter B. Prenatal diagnosis of transposition of the great vessels. Arch Mal Coeur Vaiss 2004; 97(5):580–581 (in French).

28. Kathiriya IS, Srivastava D. Left-right asymmetry and cardiac looping: implications for cardiac development and congenital heart disease. Am J Med Genet 2000; 97(4):271–279.

29. Blom NA, Ottenkamp J, Wenink AG et al. Deficiency of the vestibular spine in atrioventricular septal defects in human fetuses with Down's syndrome. Am J Cardiol 2003; 91(2):180–184.

30. Yelbuz TM, Waldo KL, Kumiski DH et al. Shortened outflow tract leads to altered cardiac looping after neural crest ablation. Circulation 2002; 106(4):504–510.

31. Jouannic JM, Fermont L, Brodaty G et al. An update on the fetal circulation. J Gynecol Obstet Biol Reprod (Paris) 2004; 33(4):291–296 (in French).

32. Jouannic JM, Picone O, Martinovic J et al. Diminutive fetal left ventricle at mid gestation associated with persistent left superior vena cava and coronary sinus dilatation. Ultrasound Obstet Gynecol 2003; 22(5):527–530.

33. Sonnesson SE, Fouron JC. Doppler velocimetry of the aortic isthmus in human fetuses with abnormal velocity waveforms in the umbilical artery. Ultrasound Obstet Gynecol 1997; 10(2):107–111.

34. Shipp TD, Bromley B, Hornberger LK et al. Levorotation of the fetal cardiac axis: a clue for the presence of congenital heart disease. Obstet Gynecol 1995; 85(1):97–102.

35. Jouannic JM, Gavard L, Fermont L et al. Sensitivity and specificity of prenatal features of physiological shunts to predict neonatal clinical status in transposition of the great arteries. Circulation 2004; 110(13):1743–1746. Epub 2004, Sep 13 (review).

36. Miyashita S, Chiba Y. Prenatal demonstration of major aortopulmonary collateral arteries with tetralogy of Fallot and pulmonary atresia. Fetal Diagn Ther 2004; 19(1):100–105.

37. Pasquini L, Tan T, Yen Ho S, Gardiner H. The implications for fetal outcome of an abnormal arrangement of the abdominal vessels. Cardiol Young 2005; 15(1):35–42.

38. Achiron R, Rotstein Z, Heggesh J et al. Anomalies of the fetal aortic arch: a novel sonographic approach to in-utero diagnosis. Ultrasound Obstet Gynecol 2002; 20(6):553–557.

39. Brown DL, Emerson DS, Shulman LP et al. Predicting aneuploidy in fetuses with cardiac anomalies: significance of visceral situs and noncardiac anomalies. J Ultrasound Med 1993; 12(3):153–161.

40. Huggon IC, Cook AC, Smeeton NC et al. Atrioventricular septal defects diagnosed in fetal life: associated cardiac and extra-cardiac abnormalities and outcome. J Am Coll Cardiol 2000; 36(2):593–601.

Chapter 2

How: technical aspects

by Jean-Eric Develay-Morice

This chapter is also covered in Part 2 of the accompanying DVD

CHAPTER CONTENTS

Ultrasound (US), which for a long time was considered as operator dependent, left little place for the images themselves. Recent legal developments in countries like France have changed this, requiring that the images taken from a US session be used in final reports concerning the patient.

> This means that all the views obtained should be of a high standard and thus able to be interpreted by different people.

To do this we must master:

- The pure US technique.
- The framing technique.
- The adaptation of the different scales of gray as it affects the physiology of our eyes.

After reviewing the physical and biologic characteristics of US we will explain those elements that fine tune our equipment allowing an examination based on, and providing, the best possible imaging.

THE PHYSICAL PRINCIPLES OF ULTRASOUND AS APPLIED TO FETAL ULTRASOUND

Tissue elasticity

The stimulation of the US probe's crystals provokes a mechanical deformation of its surface, compressing the skin gradually, and then the underlying structures. The elasticity of these deformed structures provokes a return to their original form. This new deformation brings about, on the tissues that are passed over until the probe's return, a variation of pressure which is the inverse of the initial pressure.

This is the same principle that applies to the compression of a bicycle air pump's piston when it prevents the air from leaving: the moment there is a release the piston rises. The speed of the return varies as a function of the force of the initial compression, but this is also due to the elastic characteristics of the element that is compressed, in this case, air.

> The intensity of the returning waves (and thus the quality of the image) depends on the elasticity of the tissues crossed.

Example of tissue elasticity

In this four-chamber view (Fig. 2.1), the US wave crosses tissues that present with different echogenicities in relation to their elasticity:

- Hard (e.g. a rib), which is hyperechogenic because all US is reflected, but also the waves are

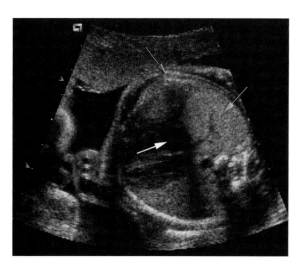

Figure 2.1 There are three different kinds of echogenicity. Anechogenic (nothing to bounce the US, which is represented in black: white arrow), hyperechogenic (most or all the US bounces off a hard structure so that it is represented in black and white as if all is reflected or absorbed: red arrow), and echogenic (intermediary hardness of the structure; the US bounces a little and is represented in gray: green arrow).

absorbed so that the structures behind cannot be visualized (red arrow).
- Liquid (e.g. a chamber), which is anechoic as there is nothing that can cause reflection so that behind this structure all the US give the impression of an augmentation of the US (blue arrow).
- Intermediary (e.g. soft tissue) (green arrow).

Reflection of ultrasound

Ultrasound acts like light: on smooth surfaces, which are sufficiently large, the reflection of the waves occurs as with a mirror. The images will be sharp if we are directly in front of them, and they will be invisible if the angle is too great. In the latter case (Fig. 2.2) the image has been reflected away from the probe, translating into an image which is anechoic.

If the surface encountered is not smooth, the resulting image will be correspondingly less sharp, such as with frosted glass, because of the "scattering" of the reflected wave (Fig. 2.3).

> We search actively for smooth surfaces that we can approach perpendicularly; this is helpful and important to remember in difficult zones.

It is important to understand that by increasing the frequency of the probe we can use the reflection, without diffusion, of a smaller surface so that intense echoes will be produced.

If by increasing the frequency we can improve the image, it is at the cost of creating a false diagnosis of hyperechogenicities (intestinal and renal—most importantly at the beginning of a pregnancy when we are most tempted to use elevated frequencies).

In the study of a smooth surface like that of the IVS, the lateral approach on the four-chamber view is preferential. The interface of the myocardium and endocardium becomes more marked and the image of the chordae more distinct than the myocardial wall. The markers are clearer, giving us a very echogenic visualization because of the endocardium, and the measure of the thickness will be more precise (IVS in the case of a gestational diabetes) (Fig. 2.4).

It is always advantageous to use perpendicular incidences in looking at interesting structures. This

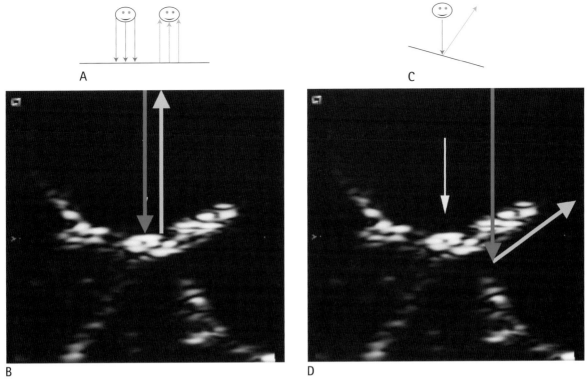

Figure 2.2   Reflection on a smooth surface can be compared to a mirror. A, B. If the US incidence is perpendicular to a smooth surface of the target, the direction of the reflected wave will be the same, thus it will return directly to the probe. This applies to the crux of the heart. C, D. If the angle is different, the entire wave is reflected away from the probe, as shown here. This also applies to the crux of the heart.

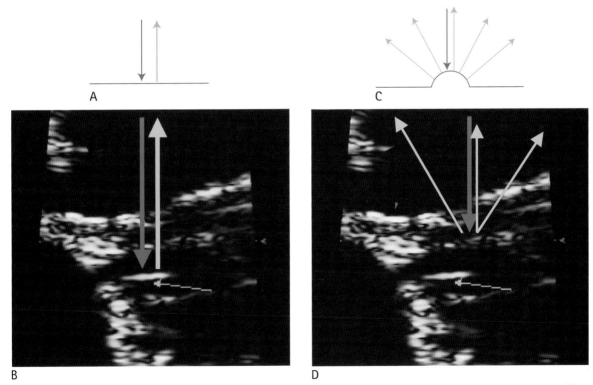

Figure 2.3   Reflection as a function of the surface of the target. A, B. If the surface is smooth, most of the wave will be reflected in the same direction. This applies to the chordae. C, D. If the surface encountered is not smooth, the resulting image will be equally less sharp with a diminished power, such as with frosted glass "scattering" a reflected wave. This applies to a jagged surface.

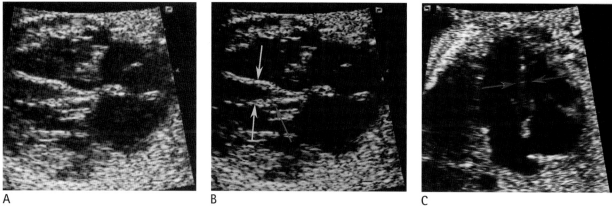

A   B   C

Figure 2.4   Cardiac application. A. In the study of a smooth surface like that of the IVS, the lateral approach on the four-chamber view is preferential. **B.** The interface of the myocardium–endocardium becomes more marked (green arrows). In this approach an important pitfall has to be avoided. The image of the chordae is more distinct than the myocardial wall allowing it to be confused with the endocardium, giving the impression of an increased thickness of the septum (red arrow). **C.** On the contrary, an apical view will limit our view of the septum (red arrow).

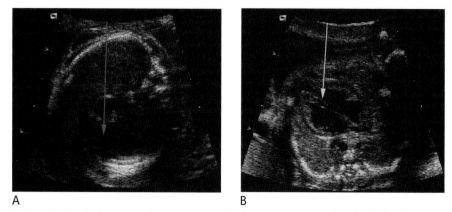

A   B

Figure 2.5   The shortest path. As an exercise we can search for the approaches that limit the distance to the fetus, positioning the left thorax in front in order to facilitate our study of the heart. **A.** This difficult path provides poor visualization of the heart, the tissue associated with the ribs causing an important attenuation (red arrow). **B.** Often after studying the spine, pressure on the back and kidneys will cause the fetus to move, allowing a better pathway with less attenuation for the examination of the heart. There will be less tissue thickness (green arrow) and fewer obstacles will greatly decrease the attenuation as well.

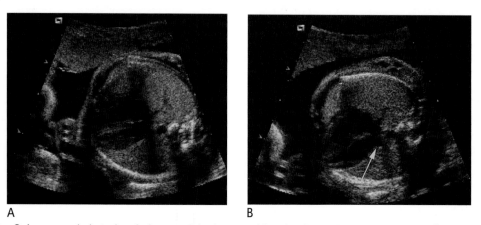

A   B

Figure 2.6   Going around obstacles. A. A cone of shadows masking the right inferior venous return (red arrow). **B.** Going around the rib to finally arrive at this vein (green arrow).

allows us to "highlight" the small smooth surfaces that would be invisible in the case of an oblique incidence.

The principle of the shortest path

The attenuation that limits exploration is in function of the quality or nature of the tissue, but also the quantity of the tissue that is passed through (Fig. 2.5).

> The path we choose is a function of the obstacles that we confront.

Going around obstacles

The more the US beam meets obstacles, the more the wave is attenuated, weakening equally the incident and reflected beam and thus finally reducing the information that can be furnished by the reflected waves. The attenuation depends on the structure of the obstacle, going from a discrete hypoechogenicity to an US wall, blocking the US and, generating impassable shadow zones, as with calcification.

Conversely, we can use these anechoic zones to facilitate the propagation of US.

In this spirit, we look for "acoustic windows" to obtain the best image, for instance using the form of a liquid near our target area to better frame the target itself (Fig. 2.6).

> We must always look for the best acoustic windows, keeping absorbent structures as far as possible outside of the trajectory of the incident wave. The very quality of our images depends directly on our ability to achieve this goal.

US can always be described as a "fight against time." There is always a compromise between the time and the quality that we are trying to obtain. (It doesn't matter if we are on vacation or in a rush, one hour always equals 60 minutes.)

We must also remember that the speed of the US propagation is independent of the constants that we may have chosen.

This speed is constant at 1560 m/s; one wave of US always has the following characteristics:

- 103 microseconds (μs) for a round trip to a depth of up to 8 cm.
- 51.5 μs for the same trajectory up to 4 cm.
- Emitting time is so short that it is negligible in relation to the reception.
- These data are absolute and invariable.

There is a limited time to emit and receive. We know that the crystal has two phases—emission and reception—which can never occur simultaneously.

At the same time we must realize that the sharpness of the final image depends on the number of points taken to form it.

Each point corresponds to a round trip of the US wave between the probe and the structure it represents.

> The image always results from a compromise between quality and frame rate (i.e. the number of images per second), which depends on our specific objectives.

To improve the frame rate, we choose those settings, from a series of parameters, which reduce useless time loss in relation to what we are looking for. These parameters are as follows:

- the surface to be explored
- the number of crystals stimulated
- the distance traveled
- the number of focus zones
- the use of color Doppler.

WHAT TAKES TIME?

The surface to be explored

The larger the surface explored and the greater the number of beamlines will vastly increase the number of pulsations to far more than what is needed. This will increase the time taken to form the image to the point that the frame rate will be greatly diminished.

It is necessary for us to limit the fields explored in our zone of interest in order to increase frame rate.

The number of crystals stimulated

This number depends on the size of the field. The greater the number of crystals stimulated, the more time we need to obtain the image. If we choose a narrow field, fewer crystals will be stimulated and this allows us to:

- Increase the number of lines per image for better definition without jeopardizing the frame rate.
- Keep the same number of lines per image in order to increase the frame rate.

Most machines allow for a lateral reduction of the field programs concerning the heart.

> In selecting a 2D zoom—and without question when we work in color—it is always preferable to choose a "box" which is higher rather than wider to increase the frame rate.

Distance traveled from the point of view of time

The deeper the field of exploration, the greater the wave trajectory. The user has no choice but to wait.

> It is therefore necessary to limit depth of field as much as possible using only what is necessary.

Some US machines limit the time of reception of echoes to those that are coming from the field being zoomed.

This gives a time advantage which can be used for increasing the frame rate and the quality of the image (by using those settings that reduce time consumption, such as the density of beamlines or the number of focal zones).

The number of focal zones

This control is often forgotten but has to be constantly adapted to the situation. This setting can optimize US since the loss of quality can be very important if the zone of interest is far from the focal zone, notably with the very high frequencies that are used in the endocavitary examination.

Something that is often overlooked—but which should be attended to when the position of the focus has been correctly adjusted—is that each sweep will be more and more precise in the small horizontal band corresponding to the focal zone. It is possible to increase this band by making several sweeps, each with a different focal band. In proceeding like this, we keep only the different focal bands from each sweep, which we will then combine to create the final images. When an image is constructed in this fashion it obviously takes more time to acquire (Fig. 2.7).

> The frame rate is divided by the number of focal zones used, which can be as high as eight or nine.

If the zone of interest is reduced and limited to the proper extent this constant can be overlooked.

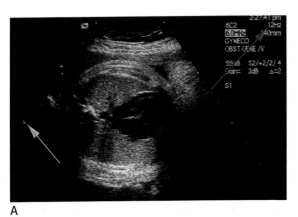
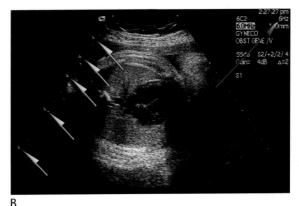

A
B

Figure 2.7   Focus. **A.** The image remains sharp *only* within the narrow band. **B.** The multiplication of narrow bands provides us with a better definition for a greater depth, but this is at the cost of lowering the frame rate. Number of focus: green arrow; frame rate: red arrow.

In doing this the US equipment will automatically adjust its maximal focal zone to the zoom which will then be entirely within this focal zone.

The use of color Doppler

The use of the Doppler effect allows us to detect the presence of movement. These then allow us to quantify direction and speed by studying the variation of the frequency undergone by the incident wave on a moving target.

Color Doppler is the greatest "time eater". Each pixel (the unit measure of each point of color) represents a pulse. Each pulse analyzes the variation in the frequency of the reflected wave provoked by the movement of each small target (whose size is only one pixel). To do this we must add the time necessary to take the 2D image.

This explains the interest in reducing, to the greatest extent possible, the surface explored in color Doppler; the time that is gained can then be used to increase image cadence or quality.

By the same mechanism, the reduction of the 2D field—even if it is less efficient than color Doppler to keep an image cadence that is satisfactory—should not be overlooked when we are studying the heart.

The time taken by Doppler in pulsed or color modes has led manufacturers to propose an independent freeze for each of these modes (in general 2D) leaving more time for what is left (in general either color and/or pulsed Doppler). Certain manufacturers refuse to use the triplex mode (2D, pulsed Doppler, and color) in order to preserve the best image quality.

THE PHYSICAL PRINCIPLES OF DOPPLER

Doppler color and time

Movement can be studied with four Doppler modes, as follows.

Continuous Doppler

This is created by variations in the frequency of reflected waves from all the tissues that are passed through by a line that is perpendicular to the probe's crystal. All these frequency variations are represented on the same curve, as if the two targets are moving in opposite directions. However, this mode is not used in obstetrics.

Pulsed Doppler

This mode allows for a limited zone of sampling along the beamline. Its correct reduction will avoid supcrimpositions of different flows. Ultrasound will arrive in a focused fashion to a very reduced quantity of tissues situated between the calipers, causing a stimulation which is very close over time and which can provoke excessive heating. In practice, this mode must be used prudently, especially during the first trimester.

Color Doppler

Pulses are distributed over a large volume and are thus much less concentrated by unit of tissue. The risk of heating is diminished, but as we have seen before, this procedure results in a distinct diminution of frame rate. In this mode information from reflected waves is transformed into colour as a function of the direction and speed of flow. Here the studied zone is a plan with many more samples than in pulsed Doppler. Each sample is seen as an individual coloured point, the totality forming a real vascular cartography.

Power Doppler

Using the same principle as color Doppler, imaging here rests on the analysis of the variation in amplitude, and not frequency. The results give us the capacity to represent flow, no matter what the direction.

These techniques follow different rules:

Incident angle

For pulsed and color Doppler, the greater part of the principles for 2D apply, except for the incident angle because these techniques are very angle dependent.

Power Doppler also uses the principles of 2D, but since it is only concerned with the variation in the amplitude of the reflected wave on a moving target (and not on its frequency), it is not angle dependent. On the other hand, it does not give information concerning direction or speed of movement.

In pulsed and color Doppler modes the angle needs to be calculated to be as close as possible within the axis of movement. It thus generates the largest variations of frequency at a constant speed.

Let's think of this another way. Imagine seeing a child throwing a ball in the direction of a car. The ball returns more quickly if the car is moving towards the child and less quickly if the car is going away. This variation of speed will be even more important if the angle of the throw is close to the angle of the axis along which the car is moving.

To see this simply in pulsed or color Doppler we consider that the principle concerning the variation of speed applies as follows:
- The wave returns more quickly if it hits a target coming towards the probe.
- The wave returns more slowly if it hits a target going away from the probe.
- These variations become optimal if the axis of the pulse is the same as that of the movement.

The physical principle corresponds to a variation in the periodicity of the reflected waves by an obstacle. This variation of periodicity allows the machine to calculate the direction and speed of movement.

Example

To search for pulmonary veins, we choose an approach to the fetus that allows us to be as close within the axis as possible in order to be able to detect the slowest flow, but at the same time allowing the best color filling (Fig. 2.8).

Pulse repetition frequency and aliasing

Pulse repetition frequency (PRF) is the frequency of pulses generated by the probe (not to be confused with the frequency of the probe, which is the characteristic of the wave that is emitted, i.e. its periodicity). A given level of PRF signifies that the examination is only accurate between a minimum and maximum flow speed.

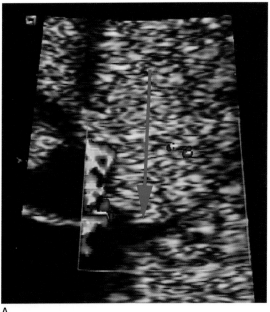
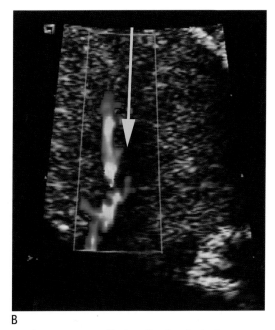

A   B

Figure 2.8   Incident angle. A. To search for pulmonary veins we choose a perpendicular allowing for better visualization of their walls (red arrow) but like this flow cannot be visualized in color Doppler. **B.** If we alter the path to be as close to the axis of flow as possible, the wall will not be seen, but flow will be optimized. This allows for the detection of the slowest flow, but will also allow the best color filling (green arrow).

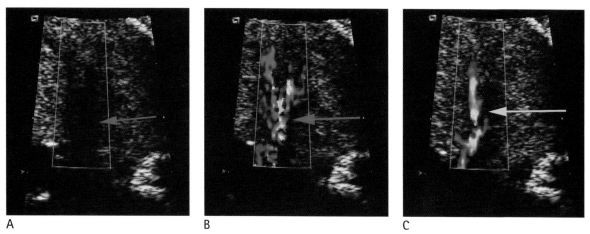

A   B   C

Figure 2.9   **PRF. A.** PRF too high: the flow is unknown. **B.** PRF too low: the flow is detected, but is too imprecise. **C.** PRF is correct: the flow is detected and indications are precise (speed, delimitation).

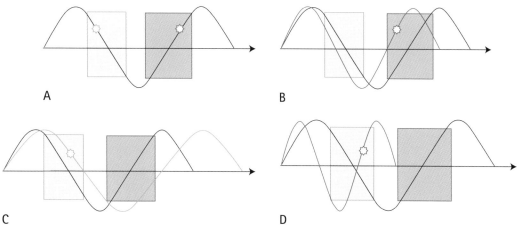

A   B

C   D

Figure 2.10   **Ultrasound wave.** The curve corresponds to the movement of one point of a target around its equilibrium point as a function of time (the green point when it returns to its equilibrium point, the red point when it is moving up). If the movement of the target changes the frequency of the US, one sinusoid apparently becomes longer. This is a function of direction and speed. PRF consists of the calculation of two time zones: one for the ascending curve (green box) and one for the descending curve (red box) when the target moves. **A.** The curve of the vibration of a point that moves on an immovable target. PRF data define the "time box" (green and red box) when the descending and ascending points (respectively green and red points) will arrive. The speed of the movement will change the period of the curve (the time to return to the equilibrium point). **B.** When the movement of the target occurs in the direction of the probe the frequency will be higher and the ascending point will come before the position it was in when the target did not move, and it will appear to "fall" more quickly, in the red box. This speed will be represented as positive. **C.** If the movement occurs in the opposite direction to the probe, the frequency will be lower so that the descending point (green point) will arrive a little later than if the target were motionless. This point will be in the green box but a little later. **D. Aliasing.** Here, the movement also occurs in the direction of the probe but its speed is faster when compared to what was predicted. The variation in the frequency will be such that the ascending point (red) will be found within the zone reserved for the descending point (green box and point). The represented color of the point cannot be differentiated by the machine so it will be calculated as a green point (a point returning to its equilibrium point) and not a red one in this box (situations shown in "C" and "D" cannot be differentiated). The subsequent interpretation of the speed will be wrongly represented as negative.

If the speed is below the minimum limit, the flow will be ignored by the device, and thus not seen.

If it is above the maximum limit, the flow will be represented by a chaotic juxtaposition of pixels going in opposite directions. It can even represent a direction that is totally the opposite of the real movement; this is the phenomena of aliasing.

This specific aspect of aliasing is well known: contiguous pixels of opposing colors. These criteria should lead us to increase the PRF until we have a homogeneous color.

On the other hand, the absence of color should lead us to lower the PRF to look for slower speeds.

> We must constantly adapt the PRF to the speed of the flow we are studying:
> * pulmonary veins: slow speed; low PRF
> * aorta: rapid flow; high PRF.

A good setting gives a homogeneous color with few pixels out of the vessel itself, thus giving a precise outline of the vessel (Fig. 2.9).

The direction of the trajectory influences the setting of the PRF concerning incident waves, which is an essential element in Doppler adjustments.

The consequence of bad settings can translate into erroneous interpretations concerning the flow direction and speed; this is also aliasing.

There is no aliasing in power Doppler because this technique gives us neither speed nor direction of flow.

The phenomenon of aliasing corresponds to the false information that is produced when reflected waves arrive outside of the period that was reserved for them. This happens most often after the departure of the next series of waves.

While the speed of an US wave is constant, the frequency of the reflected wave undergoes variations. These are provoked on the US beam by the movement of the target.

The US wave generates a sinusoid displacement of the tissues around an equilibrium point that can be represented as a curve. The frequency of the wave is represented as a function of the distance between two equilibrium points. This curve can be compared to a spring at rest attached between a wall and a car. If the car moves in the direction of the wall, the spring will compress and the coils will come closer together. The opposite will happen if the car moves away from the wall: the spring will decompress and the coils will move apart. The spring will not change if the car remains stationary. This is, more or less, the principle behind Doppler.

The curve demonstrates that at the same point an ordinate can be found which is both on the ascending and descending slope.

The US machine receives information only from points located on the curve. For every given point, its ordinate value is the same on the ascending slope as it is on the descending slope. The machine determines the slope by finding these points as a function of the time when each one of them is expected to arrive, a determination based on the supposed speed of the target. The adjustment of PRF defines this "time slot". If the real speed of the target is different from the estimation, the ascending point could arrive at the same time as the descending point, thus leading us to believe that the variation in the frequency is far more important than it really is (Fig. 2.10).

> It is advisable to adjust the PRF constantly to the speed of the examined flow. The clearest example of this "tuning" is that used to study intracardiac flow and that used for the study of the PVs.

No matter what the frequency, or the depth that is used, the emitting time is negligible in relation to the time necessary for reception.

The 3D technique

Recent and rapid technological progress has opened up new possibilities of investigation. The 3D technique is in the process of revolutionizing fetal cardiac imaging. It consists of acquiring a volume

> **!!! ATTENTION !!!**
>
> While the use of 3D makes it easier for us to acquire the right views, it can never compensate for the mediocrity of the initial images.

which is constituted by the juxtaposition of multiple US frames, acquired through a lateral mechanical sweep. This had been limited for many years to stationary targets because of the size of the acquisition which had been detrimental to image quality.

Recent advances in computer science have allowed for a considerable reduction in the time needed for acquisition, thus giving us access to volume in real time. Image quality has progressed as well, and cardiac structures can now be studied with great precision.

One of the new applications, the spatiotemporal image correlation or STIC method allows us to reconstruct the acquired views in function of the cardiac cycle, in classic color Doppler or power modes (Fig. 2.11).

Another possibility of image treatment, which is even more recent, is a mode called inversion. In this mode, hypoechogenic structures are isolated and colored, giving us a cast or mold of the cardiac chambers and vessels. This technique has the advantage of being independent of the incident angle. Contrary to Doppler, it allows the visualization of vessels undergoing widely varied speeds of flow, permitting us to have all these vessels viewed together. Moreover, as it does not use the Doppler mode, we have much more time to concentrate on finessing the image or the frame rate.

Finally one the biggest hopes for improving image quality while reducing acquisition time is the practical use of matrix volume acquisition where the mechanical sweep is replaced by an electronic one. In comparing the evolution of this technique to that of 2D, from a manual sweep of a single crystal to an electronic sweep we should expect a clear improvement in the technical quality of our examinations.

For the moment, limited to use in postnatal examinations, the exploration of the fetal heart by MRI will probably also be of great use in pathology, as soon as its resolution and acquisition speed allow it to be used efficiently.

In practice: the settings

The present day quality of US is generally sufficient to allow us to determine the normality of the heart during our first examination while keeping the same settings throughout the entire examination.

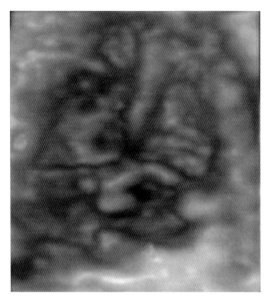

Figure 2.11   Appearance of the four-chamber view with the valves and their situation with 3D.

However, it is useful to understand what affects the image in order to know how to vary the constants to improve it.

IN PRACTICE: SETTING THE CONTROLS

The 2D settings

Zoom, focus, and gain can be modified continually, while other parameters are preset and remain constant.

Zoom

At the price of being destabilized by the new images when we first use the zoom, this function allows us to better visualize certain objects while sometimes leading us to explore structures that were not yet suspect (Fig. 2.12).

Zoom especially allows us to make adjustments targeted at the region we are studying, without letting the operator be perturbed by modifications to that image by neighboring structures.

In some US equipment the use of this parameter will only treat waves coming directly from this zone, allowing us to increase, in a substantial fashion, the image cadence, or use settings that take more time for an equivalent cadence.

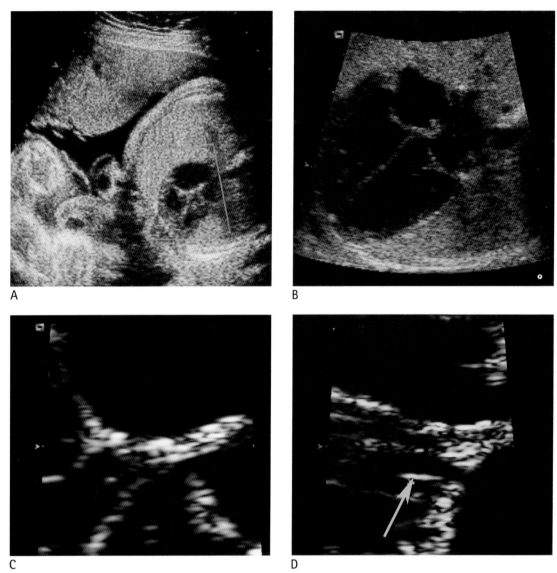

Figure 2.12   Zoom. A. The heart is too small to see the details with a poor frame rate of 20 frames per second (fps). **B.** The appropriate zoom to study the heart with a better frame rate of 40 fps. **C.** A greater zoom emphasizes structures and the different echogenicities at a frame rate of 100 fps. **D.** This zoom can lead us to unsuspected structures such as septal attachments of the tricuspid valve (green arrow) but only if we have a good trajectory. The high frame rate allows us to acquire intermediary positions of the valve during its movements.

Example of using the zoom

This is essential to the study of the heart. When we take the appropriate approach, the zoom can allow us to study previously unsuspected structures such as the crux of the heart at the septal attachments of the tricuspid valve, which would not be visible, even with the same approach if we were not using the zoom. Here we use a very specific setting, which gives preference to the interfaces and image cadence (structures whose echogenicity is very different, the heart pumping at around 145 beats per minute), but which is unusable with other organs.

Focus

Each sweep will be more precise on the small horizontal band called the focal zone, which we can move about the interest zone. Though the settings involving focus are often forgotten, we should always be sure that we have constant optimization of the placement frame (Fig. 2.13).

This problem is quickly resolved when we use a significant zoom. If the interest zone is sufficiently reduced, allowing for an important zoom, the focus settings can be forgotten because the machine will automatically place its focal zone within the zoom.

It is possible to enlarge this band by conducting several sweeps, each with a different focal zone. We then keep the focal bands of each sweep, which will eventually be juxtaposed to create the definitive image. The price we pay here is in time. The frame rate is divided by the number of focal zones used (the number of focal zones can go as high as eight or nine).

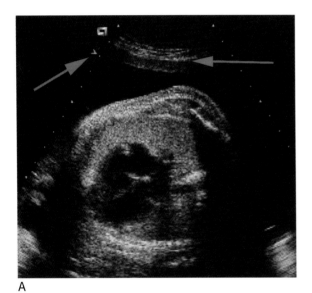

A

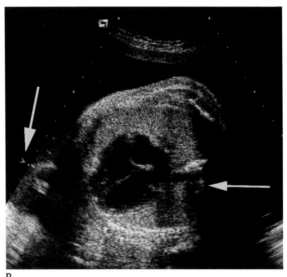

B

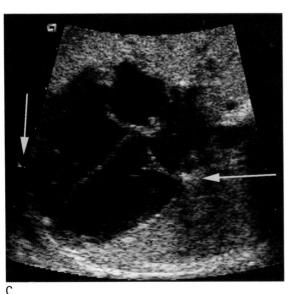

C

Figure 2.13   Focus. A. The focus is too high (red arrows) and the interest zone is less precise. B. Better definition with an appropriate position of the focus (green arrows). C. Limiting the zoom to the heart will automatically place the focus in a good position (green arrows).

For zones without movement, and when studying the entire range of a depth of field, multiply the focal zones (aortic arch and descending aorta).

For zones of fast movements and small size use one focal zone (crux of the heart).

Gain

Expressed in decibels (dB), as the logarithmic unit, it is too often elevated with the accompanying risk of "burning" the image (making it too white) and blurring the differences of echogenicity essential to the diagnosis. It should be adjusted to obtain the maximum amount of information about the studied structures, which often occurs to the detriment of the rest of the image. The characteristics of the heart are very different from other tissues, and setting the gain after using the zoom allows us to optimize the image (Fig. 2.14). Certain manufacturers have made this function automatic.

In color mode, the adjustment of gain is essential:
- *Too weak*: there would be an *absence* of flow or a feeble flow diameter, which is not the case.
- *Too elevated*: the amount of parasite signals will be multiplied, giving an image that would be difficult to interpret and showing vessel contours whose diameters are greater than that in reality.

Preset elements

Predefined on machines in the form of specific programs (for instance "general", "cardiac", or "superficial"), the precise knowledge of these settings is not essential, but can help in optimizing images or in researching precise elements such as very rapid movements like the opening of the cardiac valves.

Dynamic range

This is expressed in dB. Lowering of the dynamic hardens the image by increasing the differences between the gray levels, but it equally brings about a reduction in the quantity of grays that are available, thus the image becomes more black and white (Fig. 2.15).

This low dynamic range is not recommended when trying to differentiate a myocardial structure from pericardiac ascites because it makes the myocardium very hypoechogenic (like liquid). In case of doubt, increasing the dynamic will increase the gray scale augmenting only the myocardial echogenicity and making it visible, which will now make differentiation from ascites possible.

To study the fetal *heart*, a relatively *weak dynamic* is chosen in order to obtain clearer interfaces by diminishing the echogenicity of the blood.

To study the *myocardium*, we *raise the dynamic* to increase the sensibility of the gray scale allowing a better visualization for the study of the structures of the muscle and not simply its contours.

Frequency

Corresponding to wavelength, the higher the frequency the more precise the image will be by multiplying "mirrors" (the higher the frequency, the more that structures of smaller size act as "mirrors", generating intense echoes). At the same time attenuation increases in an exponential fashion with the thickness of the tissues that are passed through, so that the depth of field that is studied rapidly limits the zone of exploration.

The speed of conduction is independent of the frequency and has no influence on frame rate.

To simplify we begin with the highest frequency possible, whether in 2D, or color or pulsed Doppler. Then we lower it if the attenuation is too great.

The density of pulse lines per image

This adjustment is also called resolution or space-time, depending on US manufacturers.

An image is constructed based on a certain number of lines per pulse. As with frequency, the more this density is elevated, the more precise the image.

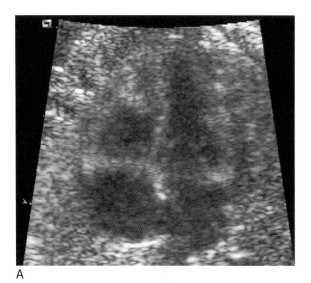

A

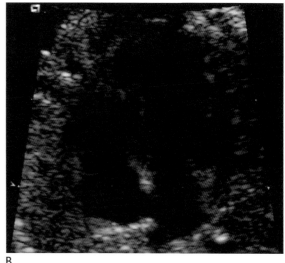

B

C

Figure 2.14   **Gain. A**. The gain is too high: gray nuances are crushed. **B**. The gain is too weak: structures such as valves with little echogenicity are ignored. **C**. Correct gain setting: an adapted gray scale is given for the zone studied.

Increasing frequency and density of lines improves the resolution.

> We seek to increase beamlines on a target that moves little.
> An efficient zoom allows an identical frame rate to increase the density of these beamlines.

Persistence

(The scale is variable depending on the specific machine.) Persistence is the superimposition of images in time which gives the "smooth" and more regular character to an image (Fig. 2.16). The heart beats at 145 times per minute and is so rapid that the images that are superimposed often have slight differences which generate a blur, such as in the visualization of the cardiac valves in their intermediary positions. This is similar to what happens when you move when taking a photograph.

> In the study of the fetal heart, *persistence eliminates blur*.

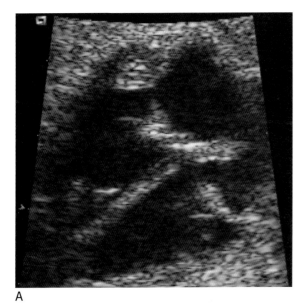

A

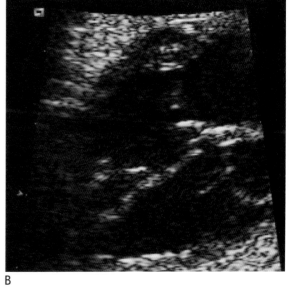

B

Figure 2.15 **Dynamics. A.** A high dynamic blocks contrast and leaves contours blurred. **B.** Lowering the dynamic makes contours more precise. **C.** Correct gain setting: an adapted gray scale is given for the zone studied so that the valve (green arrow) is particularly well seen.

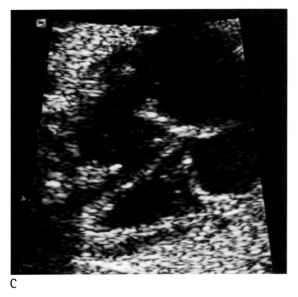

C

Contours

(The scale is variable depending on the specific machine.) This setting allows us to favor those linear elements perpendicular to the US beam (Fig. 2.17). It is especially useful in organs such as the heart with numerous interfaces (creating very intense reflective echoes) particularly with the cardiac valves. The value of this adjustment is only seen when the incidence is perpendicular.

This method is extremely useful in measuring the septum for gestational diabetes. The endocardium is smooth, the opposite of the myocardium. The echoes illustrate this, allowing us a clear limit to the septum we are measuring, but only if we have a perpendicular approach to benefit from the "mirror" effect of the smooth interfaces, i.e. by a transverse approach.

These settings will allow a good visualization of the offsetting of the atrioventricular valves at the level of the crux of the heart, with a highlighting of the oblique direction of the fibrous bridge that crosses the septum linking the mitral and tricuspid valves.

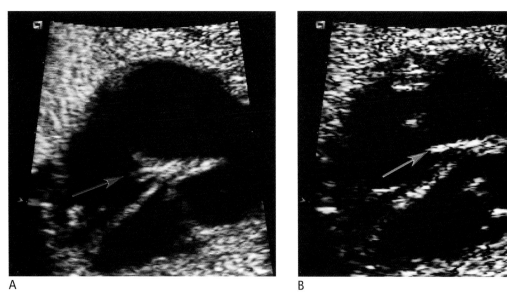

Figure 2.16   Persistence. A. Maximum persistence: the image is less hard, but produces a blur, particularly on the valves in their intermediary positions. Also, the valves will appear thickened. B. No persistence: more aggressive, the image stops every blur so that each frame become "exploitable." This setting is very important in the study of the valves and septum. Its measurement can be overestimated with the chordae being very hyperechogenic because they are parallel to the septum. This uncertainty will be cleared up by the precision of each frame, demonstrating the movements of the chordae by considering two frames. With still lower values, the cavities will appear even less echogenic with increased contrast.

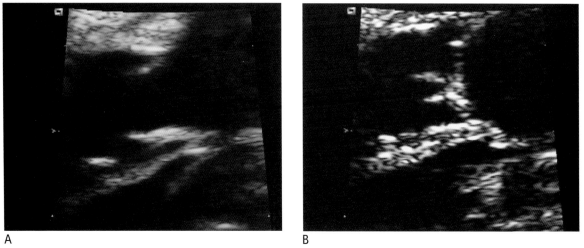

Figure 2.17   Contours. A. Few "contours" give a blur leading to problems in the study of the heart. B. The maximum use of contours gives a better visualization of the septum and valves.

Doppler settings

The same physical principles for 2D mode apply here, with special attention to the incidence of the US beam and the time factors in color Doppler where each pixel (point) corresponds to an individual roundtrip of the wave.

We must remember to optimize the size of the sampling "box" of the zone studied, to the narrowest possible, to limit the number of stimulated crystals (Fig. 2.18). This holds true whether we are in pulsed or color Doppler to gain time.

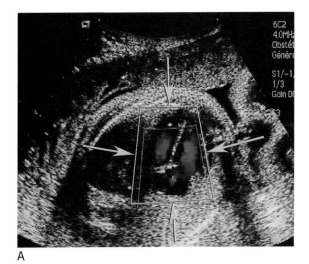

A

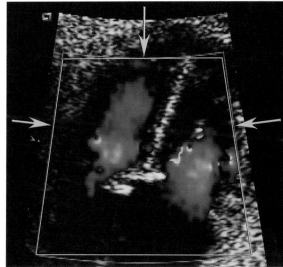

B

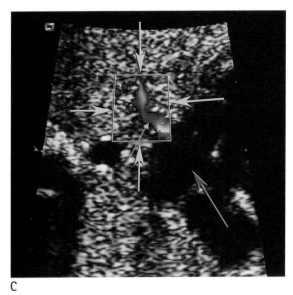

C

Figure 2.18 Zoom. A. A wide 2D window at 17 frames per second (fps). **B.** The same color "box" with a limited 2D field at 26 fps. **C.** A small 2D field with a small "box" used for the study of the pulmonary veins at 50 fps. This has the advantage of avoiding coloring the four chambers (red arrow), which would "drown" the image of the pulmonary vein.

The direction of the incident wave

In order to emphasize the variations of frequency which allow good Doppler sensitivity, as in the example presented in "Physical principles" where the child was playing with a ball, we have to be as close as possible within the axis of movement (Fig. 2.19).

Pulse repetition frequency

Pulse repetition frequency should be adapted continually to the speed of the target and the US angle so that the reception of the wave arrives in the predicted time and location reserved for it (Fig. 2.20):

● Too high: The positive speed will be considered as negative and the smallest movement will be encoded into a color which gives an image too saturated to be interpretable.
● Too low: The greater part of the vessels will be "drowning" the vessel you are looking for.

If it is too weak, flow will be ignored.

For studying the heart, the PRF should be set at the maximum to search only the most rapid flow. On the other hand, it should be much lower to reduce the "box" when studying the pulmonary veins.

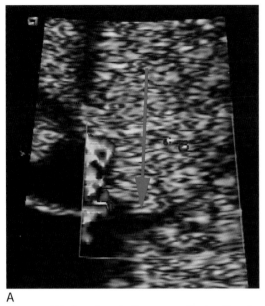
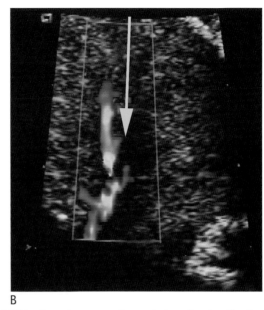

A   B

Figure 2.19 US direction. A. The perpendicular direction of US in the pulmonary veins optimizes the visualization of their walls in 2D (red arrow) but leads us to believe that there is an absence of flow. **B.** By simply modifying the incident angle it is possible to make the vein's flow appear (green arrow), as the "walls" of the veins are made to disappear.

Color gain

The setting for color gain is often forgotten. It is preferable to make this adjustment last after having selected the zone of exploration and the PRF (Fig. 2.21).

If the gain is:

- Too weak, we will have the impression that there is no flow and we could underestimate the flow diameter, even the size of the vessel.
- Too high, we will have a number of parasites that will mask the flow. Filling will appear blurred, giving the impression of a flow diameter, and thus a vessel size, greater than in reality.

APPLICATION TO THE EXAMINATION OF THE FETAL HEART

The echo-structure

The echogenic gradient of cardiac tissue is particularly important, linked to the differences in cardiac tissue blood, but also because of the structural differences of the various cardiac tissues themselves.

- The myocardium is a tissue which is not very dense, made by fibers going off in every direction, and thus, for US, it is not angle dependent.
- Valvular tissue and chordae are, on the contrary, very dense tissues, of a fibrous nature having a single direction generating an important mirroring effect, leaving them very angle dependent for US examination.
- The endocardium is an intermediary tissue for US reflection. A perpendicular approach can differentiate it from the myocardium, a characteristic which is particularly interesting in the estimation of the septum's thickness in a diabetic pathology.

The position of the fetal heart

The fetal heart is found lying flat on a horizontally viewed diaphragm, surrounded by the ribs. The pathways to approach it are thus narrow in a fetus whose position is variable (head, breech, transverse, etc.) and in almost constant movement. All of these elements taken together require that we have an excellent understanding of the position and anatomy of the heart in order to determine, in advance,

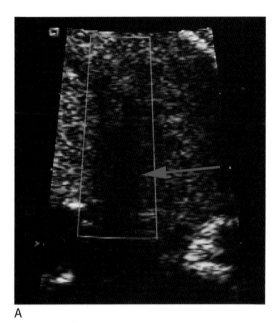

A

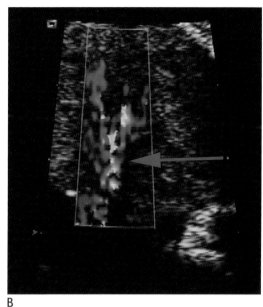

B

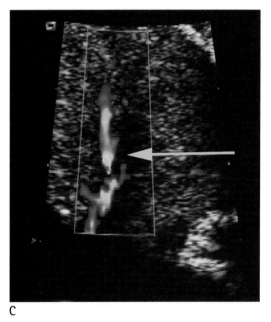

C

Figure 2.20   **PRF. A.** PRF is too high for the flow so it is ignored (red arrow). **B.** PRF is too low for the flow, causing aliasing. Most of the color is red, representing a false direction for these veins, with some blue side by side, which represents an opposite direction (red arrow). We can only conclude that there is a flow. **C.** PRF is well set giving a homogeneous flow in blue representing the correct direction (green arrow), with a clear indication of the speed.

the approach path to take which will favor each of our reference views.

The movements

The target, i.e. the heart, moves quickly and instinctively we must follow these movements. Not only does our target move quickly, but the position of the fetus itself constantly varies.

- The heart is beating at an average of 145 beats per minute, necessitating that we favor frame rate, especially for the kinetics of the valves.
- The respiratory movements sometimes force us to place ourselves in the correct position in relation to the fetus, and then wait patiently until the structures we want to study pass before the US window to be captured.

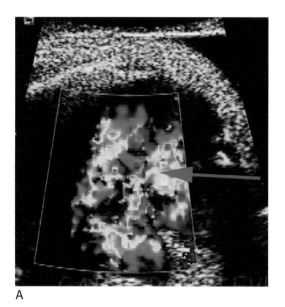

A

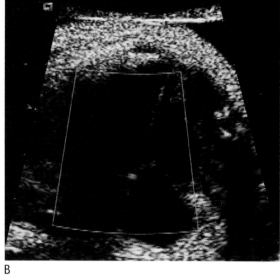

B

Figure 2.21   Gain. A. The gain is too high, the image artifact "burns" the true flow. **B.** The gain is too weak and the flow is overlooked. **C.** The gain is correct, visualizing the flow with a good filling of the four chambers.

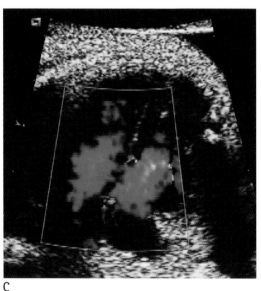

C

● There are certain movements of the fetus that we can use by knowing when to wait, or even by provoking them ourselves, causing subsequent changes in the position of the fetus which will be more favorable for the view we are looking for.

The aim of the US specialist should be to see the elements directly from the front taking great care to avoid "wave eaters" that precede the target, always placing ourselves in the axis of movement of the Doppler.

Further reading

Arbeille P. Mise au point 2003 sur les risques d'effets biologiques par échographie, Doppler pulsé et couleur in SFAUMB 2003; www.sfaumb.org

Chaoui R, Hoffmann J, Heling KS. Three-dimensional (3D) and 4D color Doppler fetal echocardiography using spatio-temporal image correlation (STIC). Ultrasound Obstet Gynecol 2004; 23(6):535–545.

Kremkau FW. Diagnostic ultrasound: principles and instruments, 5th edn. Philadelphia: W.B. Saunders Co. Ltd; 1998.

Kremkau FW, Taylor KJ. Artifacts in ultrasound imaging. J Ultrasound Med 1986; 5(4):227–237.

Lee W, Goncalves LF, Espinoza J, Romero R. Inversion mode: a new volume analysis tool for 3-dimensional ultrasonography. J Ultrasound Med 2005; 24(2):201–207.

Chapter 3

How: anatomic–ultrasound correlations; 3 steps, 10 key points

by Catherine Fredouille

 This chapter is also covered in Part 3 of the accompanying DVD

Just as we would do before any clinical examination we begin by taking a medical history and through our questioning look to uncover several important points, including:

- Family history of CHD. Known congenital cardiopathies in the parents or siblings,[1] as well as unexplained neonatal deaths in relatives.
- Risk factors. Administration of lithium or an anti-epileptic (even in the case of treatment by folic acid), diabetes,[2] or phenylketonuria. Remember that the consumption of alcohol is rarely obvious.[3]
- The presence of a known normal karyotype. If there is a request to assess nuchal translucency (NT), the NT value is of great importance—an NT of 6 mm is of greater diagnostic value than that of 3 mm—as its discovery during the first trimester correlates with the highest frequency of cardiopathies,[4] as well as genetic syndromes.[5]

After taking this history we then verify cardiac architecture in 3 steps and 10 key points. These have been designed to exclude all the important pathologies that can be seen in the fetus.

Using this method, the practice of an ultrasound (US) examination can be compared to reading a large book (Figs 3.1–3.3).

1. The transabdominal diameter (TAD) is the cover.
2. After several pages of introduction we reach the inlet chapter. Of course we can read each of the pages of this chapter, but all the important information can be found summarized on *one* page. This page is the "optimal" four-chamber

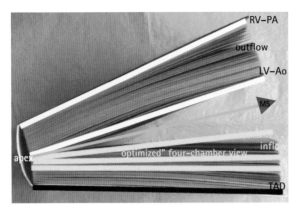

Figure 3.1 Left view with the "book" cover open.

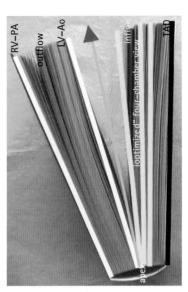

Figure 3.2 Open "book", vertical view.

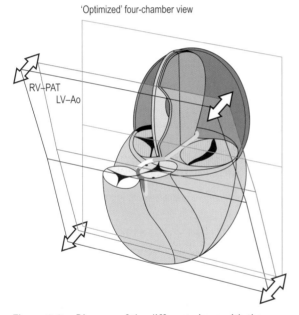

Figure 3.3 Diagram of the different views with the heart seen vertically.

view, which we will introduce later and define how you can obtain it.

3. This book has also certain "dangerous" pages for the fetal US practitioner. Situated at the junction between the chapters on inlet and outlet, where the membranous septum is explored, here we see the location of the small ventricular septal defects (VSDs) which we can clearly differentiate from VSDs of the inlet septum or outlet septum. The VSDs of the membranous septum—translated clinically by heart murmurs—are the most frequent pathologies in pediatric cardiology.

Prenatally, aside from their chance association with a pathologic context, finding these small VSDs, which are strictly confined within the membranous septum, will have no great consequence during the entire pregnancy, except prematurely worrying the parents about a problem, which in most cases, will diappear spontaneously in early infancy. Their discovery in the postnatal pediatric examination will not affect their prognosis either.

4. Past this "zone to avoid", the outlet chapter needs to be consulted thoroughly—start to finish, up and down, right to left, even diagonally—to be fully understood.

At the end of this examination the US specialist will be able to attach images of these normal findings to the medical dossier of the patient.

In the case of an anomaly, the specialist will do his or her best to produce images in several views. This provides the opportunity to eliminate those false images which are always possible. In the case of the discovery of a cardiac pathology by the first physician, or during the course of the first examination, the most complete morphological examination should be made before referring the patient to a more specialized US practitioner of reference. In the case of an isolated cardiopathy, a pediatric cardiologist should be consulted to confirm the diagnosis, and above all, the prognosis.

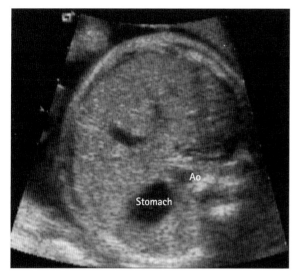

Figure 3.4   Ultrasound TAD view. Note the stomach and aorta on the left.

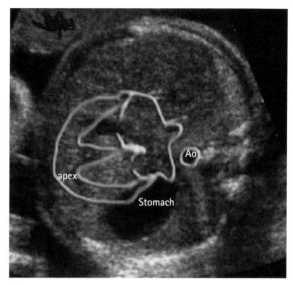

Figure 3.5   The same view as in Figure 3.4 with a superimposed diagram of the heart at the level of the four-chamber view. Note the aorta and apex on the left.

FIRST STEP. VERIFICATION OF THE POSITION: 2 KEY POINTS

- **Point 1** This concerns the elements of lateralization. Here we look to the right of the fetus for the gall bladder and the inferior vena cava (IVC). To the left of the fetus we find the stomach (Fig. 3.4) at the abdominal level, and then we look at the apex of the heart at the thoracic level (Fig. 3.5) with always only one vessel in front and to the left of the spine, and then behind the LA, the descending aorta.
- **Point 2** This relates to the axis of the heart. The apex of the heart is normally directed towards the left and the interventricular septum (IVS), which represents this axis, making an angle of about 45° (Fig. 3.6) with the anteroposterior axis.[6]

In practice

These two points can be confirmed by passing between the TAD and the four-chamber view by taking the "elevator" (Fig. 3.7).

After determining the fetal position (cephalic or breech presentation, the position of the back), we perform the TAD view. We see to the left of the spine the descending aorta with, in front of it, the stomach, and in the center a part of the umbilical vein. To the right, behind the gall bladder, the IVC

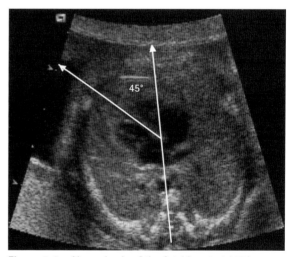

Figure 3.6   Normal axis of the fetal heart at 45° in relation to the anteroposterior axis.

is situated in front of the right adrenal. In the transverse views, a good visualization of the larger part of the distal rib(s) (as proximally the US beam passes between two ribs) confirms the axial character of the fetal view. In apical incidences we try to view two lateral complete ribs.

Once the localization has been verified, the view is stable, and the TAD image is taken, we take the

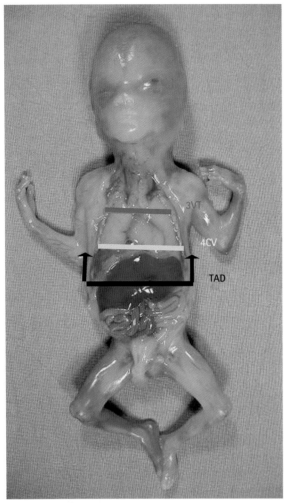

Figure 3.7   The fetus seen from the front showing the levels of the different views. The black arrows show the TAD/four-chamber view translation. 3VT, three vessels and trachea view; 4CV, four-chamber view.

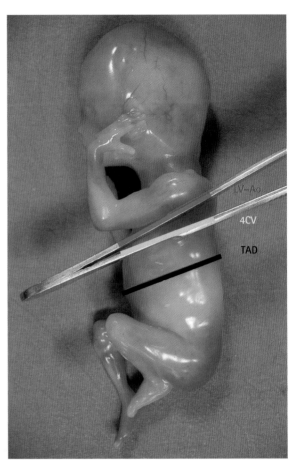

Figure 3.8   The fetus seen in profile showing the levels of the different views. Note the acute angle between the four-chamber view/LV–Ao.

"elevator" and do a cephalic translation (Fig. 3.8) along the two vascular axes which constitute the aorta and the IVC. Several intercostal spaces higher, we arrive at the level of the optimal four-chamber view with its reference points: the apex and the two inferior pulmonary veins (PVs). In paying particular attention to the IVC during this translation, we note that it receives the subhepatic veins, and then crosses the diaphragm and emerges into the right atrium (RA) in contact with the foramen ovale (FO).

Verification of lateralization

Position of the organs

The gall bladder is to the right, the stomach and the heart to the left. It is not enough to see these two organs on the same side: you must ensure that you are in fact looking at the left side of the fetus. To do this, we use our Situs Wheel, created for the US operator who works directly in front, facing the patient (Fig. 3.9).

The outer circle of the Situs Wheel's outer ring is used to date the pregnancy. The Wheel is composed of two sides, which correspond to fetal presentation (cephalic or breech). In front of each fetal position, we see a diagram of the four-chamber

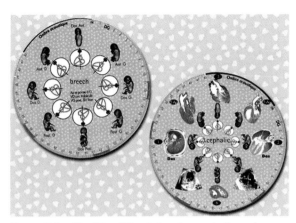

Figure 3.9   The Situs Wheel showing cephalic and breech presentations.

view corresponding to the orientation for this specific position. In comparing the diagram situated directly in front of the position of the fetus being examined with that of the screen image, we can verify the lateralization. In this way we ensure that the stomach and heart, seen to be situated on the same side, are definitely on the left side of the fetus. In fact, for the same position of the fetal back, depending on whether the fetus is in a cephalic or breech presentation, the image of the four-chamber view is mirrored on the screen and the Wheel. Comparing the US image and the diagram on the Wheel with the presentation of the position of the fetal back allows us to eliminate complete situs inversus.

Vessel position

The abdominal aorta is situated in front and to the left of the spine. The IVC (Fig. 3.10) has been located at the abdominal level, more to the front of the right kidney. The gall bladder is included in the right lobe of the liver, which is normally very large in the fetus. In left isomerisms of visceroatrial heterotaxia (VAH), the suprarenal part of the IVC can be missing. There is then seen a voluminous azygos venous return, which forms a large parallel vessel (Fig. 3.11) alongside the aorta, before crossing the posterior part of the thorax to reach the superior vena cava (SVC).[7]

Axis of the heart   The apex of the heart is normally directed towards the left, its axis represented by the IVS (see Fig. 3.5). This axis normally makes an angle close to 45° with the anteroposterior axis.[6] As in anatomy, where it is represented by the position of the anterior interventricular coronary artery, which passes over the IVS, it is an excellent measure of the size, and thus the balance, between the ventricular chambers of the inlet.

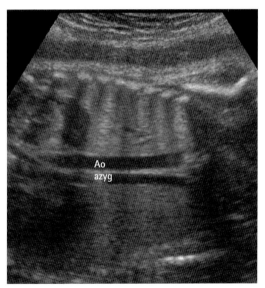

Figure 3.11   Two parallel vessels in a sagittal thoracic–abdominal view in the case of a pathology (visceroatrial heterotaxia).

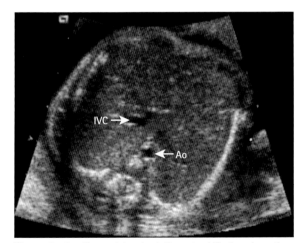

Figure 3.10   Transabdominal diameter US view. Location of the aorta and the IVC.

SECOND STEP. VERIFICATION OF THE INLET: 4 KEY POINTS

We will verify the following:

- **Point 3** That the heart is placed flat on the diaphragm, anchored to the lungs by the inferior PVs.
- **Point 4** There are four chambers (simply said, exactly four: neither three nor five).
- **Point 5** The chambers are contractile, balanced, and concordant.
- **Point 6** The crux of the heart is composed of two anuli that are permeable and offset.

In practice

Point 3: the heart is attached by the inferior PV

This finding is one of the keys in obtaining the optimal four-chamber view (Fig. 3.12). As for the TAD, seeing one—or even two—complete ribs guarantees the axial character of this view: the heart flat on the diaphragm (Fig. 3.13).

The localization of the two inferior PVs and the apex (Fig. 3.14) is ideal in confirming the view used in studying the crux of the heart. Its axial character is confirmed by seeing at least one complete rib (Fig. 3.15).

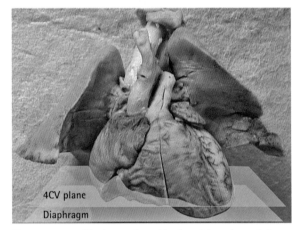

Figure 3.13 The heart–lung block—with a view of the four chambers which is parallel to the plane of the diaphragm.

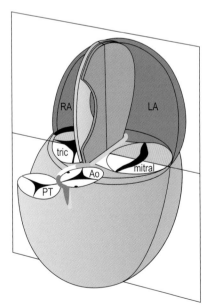

Figure 3.12 Diagram of the four-chamber view on the "verticalized" heart.

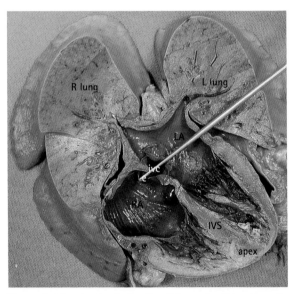

Figure 3.14 Anatomic "optimal" four-chamber view of cardiac–pulmonary block. The probe passes to the Eustachian valve to the right and the flap valve to the left.

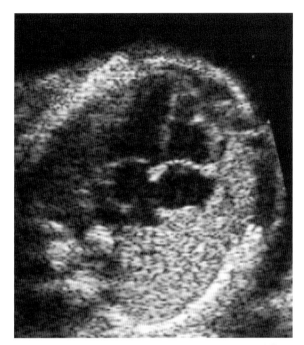

Figure 3.15 The "optimal" four-chamber thoracic US view on which we can see the 4 key points, with the ribs as reference points.

After zooming we will keep the sequence in cine-loop of this optimal view. It is through this that we can then study (and save) the images of the 4 key points concerning the inlet.

Points 4 and 5: the four chambers should be balanced and concordant

Once the optimal view has been obtained, we can see (in the LA where the inferior PV arrives) the normal motion of the FO flap valve directed by the oxygenated blood flow from the IVC (Figs 3.16 and 3.17). The other atrium is the RA. Each atrium should be concordant with its respective ventricle: the RA with the RV, just as the LA is with the LV. Anteriorly, the RV is situated behind the sternum and is recognizable by its coarse trabeculations which leave it relatively echogenic. The LA communicates with the LV and must form the apex of the heart. The left side of the IVS should be very smooth. This chamber is clearly less echogenic than that of the RV.

Figure 3.16 Anatomic view of the "optimal" four-chamber view.

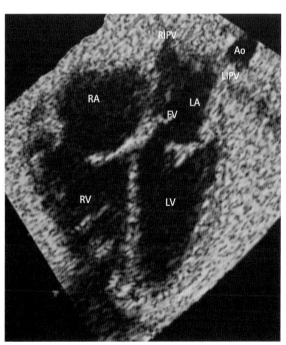

Figure 3.17 Ultrasound view of the "optimal" four-chamber view.

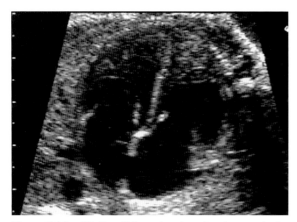

Figure 3.18 "Optimal" four-chamber view in an apical incidence with the valves open.

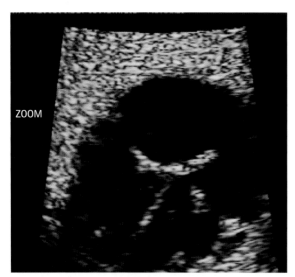

Figure 3.19 The crux of the heart seen with a zoom using an approach perpendicular to the insertion of the tricuspid.

Point 6: the two permeable and offset atrioventricular valves

The permeability (Fig. 3.18) of the mitral and tricuspid valves is dynamically explored. It is done in this manner because we can better observe the offsetting of the atrioventricular valves in systole by approaching tricuspid insertion in a direction perpendicular to that insertion (Fig. 3.19).[8]

The fetal heart examination *must* begin at the abdominal level.
The first and second steps are studied by using short sequences of cineloops taken during the TAD view (through to the optimal four-chamber view), all of the *highest quality*.
The image from the optimal four-chamber view should be clear and evident, allowing any specialist to confirm the key points at any time afterwards (Fig. 3.20).

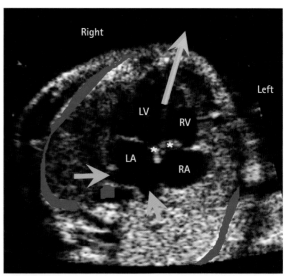

Figure 3.20 Verifying the four-chamber US view. The position (apex and aorta to the left with an axis of 45°) and the inlet (four balanced and concordant chambers with two anuli that are permeable and offset). Note the complete ribs.

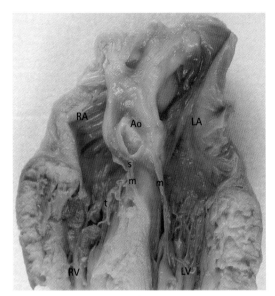

Figure 3.21   Anatomic four/five-chamber view passing through the atrioventricular zone of the membranous septum.

THIRD STEP. VERIFICATION OF THE OUTLET: 4 KEY POINTS

These key points are often difficult to verify in this order; but they all must be seen to confirm normal architecture.

- **Point 7** The two outlet chambers are balanced and separated by a septum in alignment. We should also check the septal–aortic continuity and the mitral–aortic continuity.

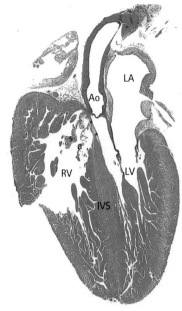

Figure 3.23   Histologic four/five-chamber view passing through the interventricular zone of the membranous septum (between the two asterisks). Note the two leaflets of the tricuspid. a, anterior leaflet; s, septal leaflet.

- **Point 8** The two vessels are crossed and superimposed.
- **Point 9** Their size is balanced and they are concordant.
- **Point 10** The aortic arch is regular.

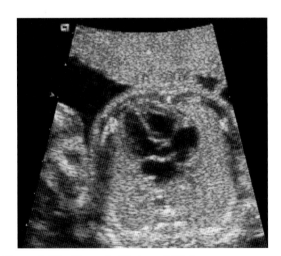

Figure 3.22   Thoracic US view of LV–Ao.

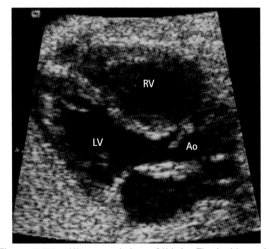

Figure 3.24   Ultrasound view of LV–Ao. The incidence is perpendicular to the wall making it appear echogenic.

In practice

By multiplying the axial, sagittal, and coronal views of the fetus we can verify these 4 key points.

Point 7: the verification of septal– and mitral–aortic continuity

In "opening" the "book" and taking care not to venture into the MS zone (Fig. 3.21), which we achieve by jumping from the optimal four-chamber view to the LV–Ao view, we can follow the trajectory of the LV–Ao which is normally tortuous. (Fig. 3.22) The MS is very thin (Fig. 3.23)

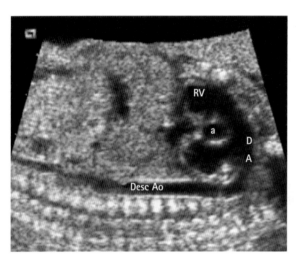

Figure 3.25 Ultrasound view of the ductus arteriosus (DA).

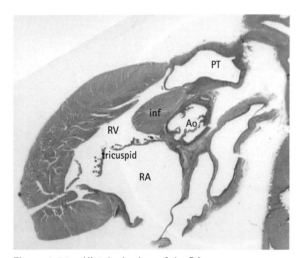

Figure 3.26 Histologic view of the DA.

and can perhaps be mistaken for a defect in an apical view. To avoid any error, we must take a perpendicular image of the ring (Fig. 3.24). Outlet VSDs are usually large and particularly well seen here because they are due to the absence of a closing in the upper part of the muscular outlet IVS. There is a loss of the fibrous–muscular continuity with the aorta, which is found to be overriding and misaligned. The other wall of the aorta is in fibro–fibrous continuity to the aortic mitral leaflet (see Figs 1.40 and 1.41).

Point 8: crossing of the two vessels

Statically we use the view called the ductus arteriosus (DA), which is a sagittal view that is slightly oblique (Fig. 3.25). It allows us to observe, on the same view, the two vessels cut at the level of their leaflets to see if the orifices are contiguous and orthogonal. However, strict criteria need to be used: the image must be taken at the level of the valvular leaflets and should be confirmed by seeing the echogenic valvular points in the lumen of each vessel. The anulus of the anterior PT is seen cut on a longitudinal plane. The aortic anulus is seen cut transversally at its origin in the center of the heart. At the level of the histologic view (Figs 3.25 and 3.26), passing by the IVC, one should see clearly,

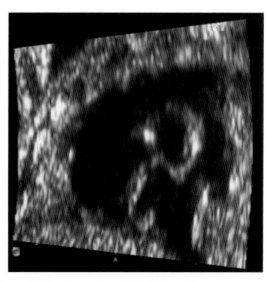

Figure 3.27 The sagittal RV–PA view allows us to compare the diameters of these vessels and confirm the concordance.

in the form of an echogenic arc, the anterior tricuspid valve equally in continuity with the aortic anulus (while the tricuspid and the valve of the PT are at a distance, separated by the infundibulum) (Fig. 3.27).

Dynamically, visualization is accomplished by passing from the RV–TP to the LV–Ao special views (Figs 3.28 and 3.29). This is often difficult to approach apically so we try to obtain the intersection of the oblique views as near as possible to the coronal views of the heart. We call this the *guédoufle* view (in reference to the distinctive oil and vinegar bottle; see Fig. 1.48). This view of the ventricles is accomplished at the level of the papillary muscles. The LV is recognized by its rounded form and the presence of these two papillary muscles. The RV, with its trabeculated structure, forms a "crescent moon" surrounding the LV. Unlike the LV, only one papillary muscle is present in the lumen of the RV. Anterior to the RV, the PT moves in a short, straight trajectory towards the descending aorta, posteriorly and to the left. The aorta, coming out of the rounded ventricle with two papillary muscles, has a tortuous trajectory, whose beginning is quasi-perpendicular to that of the PT. These two vessels are at first contiguous but then move in an initial direction that is quasi-perpendicular, finally joining at the level of the descending aorta.

The trajectory of the PT to the descending aorta is short, straight and anteroposterior. That of the aorta takes an arched pathway.

Point 9: balance and concordance of the vessels

In all of the previously described views it is important to appreciate the relative diameters of the great vessels. These vessels are known to be very similar in size, with a small superiority in diameter to that of the PT over the aorta, due to differences in the flow that passes through them. The concordance is confirmed by the exit of the PT from the RV, which is situated behind the sternum (Fig. 3.30). Its trajectory is anteroposterior, almost in a straight line. The aorta begins in the LV and the center of the heart (see Fig. 3.24). Taking a tortuous trajectory, it rejoins the same vessel, the descending aorta.

The size of these vessels can be appreciated in different ways, either at the level of the DA view for the anuli, or at the level of the three-vessel view for the ducts (Fig. 3.31).[9] This last view allows us to pay special attention to the junction between the aortic arch and the descending aorta. It is at this level that we can appreciate the size of the aortic isthmus, the zone implicated in the development of most coarctations occurring after the postnatal closure of the DA.

While the verification of normal cardiac architecture does not require the systematic use of

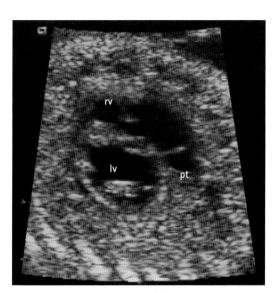

Figure 3.28   *Guédoufle* view of RV–TP.

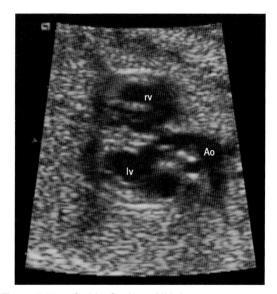

Figure 3.29   *Guédoufle* view of LV–Ao.

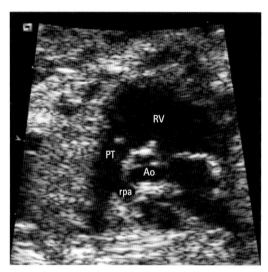

Figure 3.30 Ultrasound concordance on the small axis of RV-PA.

Doppler, the verification of the direction of flow of the arches in the three-vessel view in Doppler mode (Figs 3.31 and 3.32) gives us an extra degree of normality; inverted flow at this level is always pathologic.[10]

Point 10: regular aortic arch

Paradoxically this is easier to see in a fetus from the back than from the front. The view of the aortic arch is obtained parasagittally, passing to the left of the fetal spine. From the point where the aorta emerges, from its shape and the size of its anulus, we can gather diverse information. A normal aortic arch begins in the center of the heart in the form of a candy cane, and from its arch three vessels emerge (Fig. 3.33).

You must confirm the diameter of the entire arch globally on a parasagittal view (Figs 3.33 and 3.34), especially at the level of the aortic isthmus between the left common carotid artery (LCCA) and the junction of the DA with the descending aorta.[11] We also try to check (with the three-vessel view) the horizontal aorta between the right common carotid artery (RCCA) and the LCCA. In the case of an anomaly of the aortic arch, a stenosis, or an interruption, the presence of a VSD—often difficult to discern but important to confirm—should be investigated. This is done in order to diagnose a syndrome of coarctation or an IAA. Cases such as these belong to the CT spectrum, and abnormality of the aorta is always associated with an outlet VSD. Complementary research of a 22q11 deletion should be requested.

The third step requires static and dynamic studies obtained using complementary views.

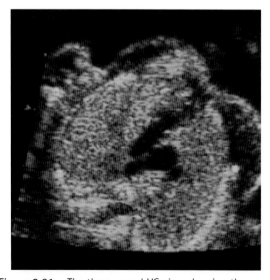

Figure 3.31 The three-vessel US view showing the relative sizes of the arches.

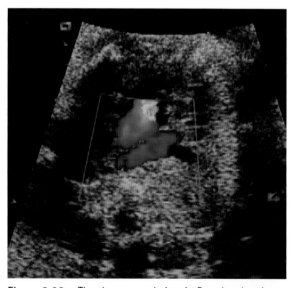

Figure 3.32 The three-vessel view in Doppler showing that flow is in the same direction.

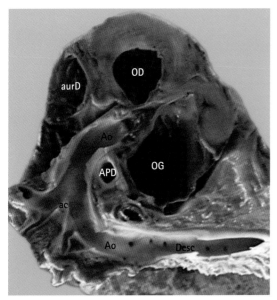

Figure 3.33   Anatomic view of the aortic arch.

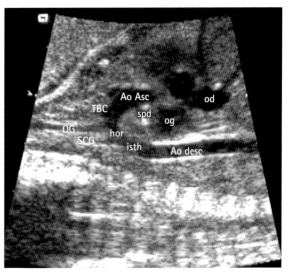

Figure 3.34   Ultrasound view of the aortic arch.

References

1. Oberhansli I, Extermann P, Jaggi E, Pfizenmaier M. Fetal echocardiography in pregnancies of women with congenital heart disease – clinical utility and limitations. Thorac Cardiovasc Surg 2000; 48(6):323–327.

2. Chung CS, Myrianthopoulos NC. Factors affecting risks of congenital malformations. II. Effect of maternal diabetes on congenital malformations. Birth Defects Orig Artic Ser 1975; 11(10):23–38.

3. Loser H, Pfefferkorn JR, Themann H. Alcohol in pregnancy and fetal heart damage. Klin Padiatr 1992; 204(5):335–339. In German.

4. Bahado-Singh RO, Wapner R, Thom E et al. Elevated first-trimester nuchal translucency increases the risk of congenital heart defects. Am J Obstet Gynecol 2005; 192(5):1357–1361.

5. Souka AP, von Kaisenberg CS, Hyett JA et al. Increased nuchal translucency with normal karyotype. Am J Obstet Gynecol 2005; 192(4):1005–1021. Erratum in: Am J Obstet Gynecol 2005; 192(6):2096.

6. Shipp TD, Bromley B, Hornberger LK et al. Levorotation of the fetal cardiac axis: a clue for the presence of congenital heart disease. Obstet Gynecol 1995; 85(1):97–102.

7. Pasquini L, Tan T, Yen Ho S, Gardiner H. The implications for fetal outcome of an abnormal arrangement of the abdominal vessels. Cardiol Young 2005; 15(1):35–42.

8. Vettraino IM, Huang R, Comstock CH. The normal offset of the tricuspid septal leaflet in the fetus. J Ultrasound Med 2002; 21(12):1386. Author reply: 1386.

9. Yoo SJ, Lee YH, Cho KS. Abnormal three-vessel view on sonography: a clue to the diagnosis of congenital heart disease in the fetus. Am J Roentgenol 1999; 172(3)825–830.

10. Vinals F, Heredia F, Giuliano A. The role of the three vessels and trachea view (3VT) in the diagnosis of congenital heart defects. Ultrasound Obstet Gynecol 2003; 22(4):358–367.

11. Sonnesson SE, Fouron JC. Doppler velocimetry of the aortic isthmus in human fetuses with abnormal velocity waveforms in the umbilical artery. Ultrasound Obstet Gynecol 1997; 10(2):107–111.

Chapter 4

How: conducting the examination and its pitfalls

by Jean-Eric Develay-Morice

 This chapter is also covered in Part 4 of the accompanying DVD

CHAPTER CONTENTS

In this chapter we further develop our method which allows us to say, that the fetal heart is normal, proving this by our choice of the criticial reference images. This point also has important medicolegal implications.[1]

TAKING THE HISTORY

We begin by taking a family history of congenital heart disease (CHD) in the current or previous pregnancies. This information should not be neglected and will direct us in the way we conduct the examination itself. Even though the study of the crux of the heart should be systematic, the knowledge of a nuchal translucency or of the triple test could place this particular type of pregnancy in a risk category, with the subsequent need to more clearly demonstrate the normal alignment of the atrioventricular valves. This is the case in diabetes, where the septal thickness needs to be measured by precise criteria.

For those who practice obstetric ultrasound (US), the heart is considered the most difficult organ to investigate.

Our examination of the heart begins with the transabdominal (TAD) view. If we are experienced and comfortable in doing this we have the foundation for what follows—a cranial translation of the probe from the TAD position will provide an excellent review of the state of the entire heart, and in most instances will also allow us to appreciate the normality of the heart.

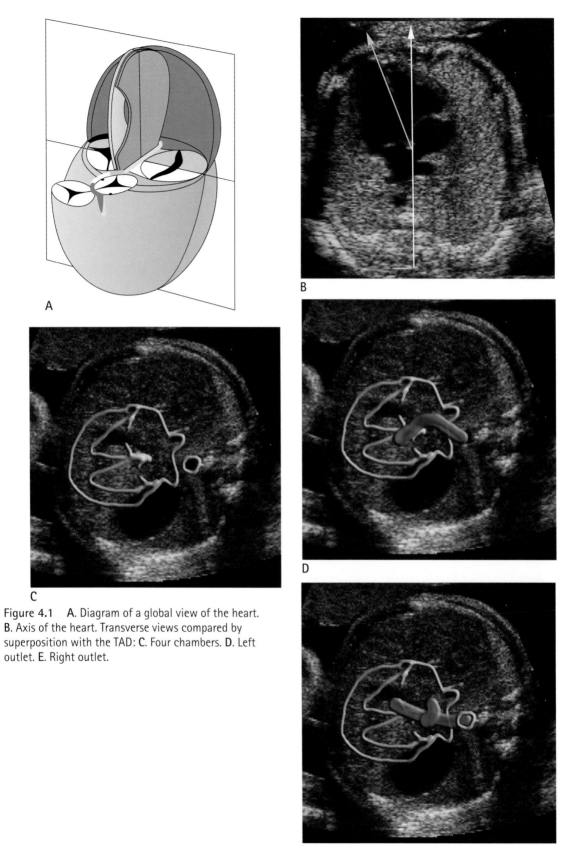

Figure 4.1 A. Diagram of a global view of the heart. B. Axis of the heart. Transverse views compared by superposition with the TAD: C. Four chambers. D. Left outlet. E. Right outlet.

The fetal heart examination is less a problem of acquisition than to recognize different structures, requiring a precise knowledge of the positioning of each element we study.

The main difficulty in the acquisition of reference views in studying the heart comes from the skeletal cage that surrounds it. We must use our knowledge to avoid bony obstacles such as the ribs, the spine, and even sometimes limbs, which will get in between the probe and the thorax. If the fetal position makes studying the heart too difficult—e.g. when the fetal back is anterior—we should not hesitate to study other, more accessible, organs such as the kidneys. In most cases, the fetus will move so that later in the examination we will have a better position for studying the heart.

Let us first look at the position of these views compared with the TAD reference scan and then examine sagittal and transversal views of the fetus (Figs 4.1 and 4.2).

If we discipline ourselves to use a good quality abdominal view the essential elements of heart US will consist of moving in the direction of the fetal head by a movement of the wrist.

A FAST GLANCE

Before going into the details of the examination we begin by taking a quick preliminary look round the entire area. This is done to avoid finding unexpected major cardiac anomalies later on, well after the morphological examination is underway. It is advisable to make these observations at the very beginning of the examination.

We move upwards and parallel towards the cephalic pole, beginning from the transverse abdominal view (after lateralization, with the stomach on the left), and then pass to the four-chamber view, from this point rapidly continuing along the beginning of the aorta to arrive at the pulmonary trunk (PT). Continuing the movement, we see the horizontal portion of the aortic arch using the three-vessel view. We can, with great benefit, do the same examination in the color mode (Figs 4.3 and 4.4).

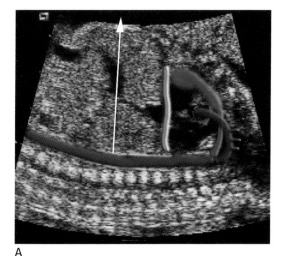

A

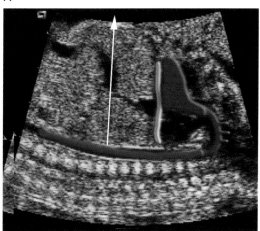

B

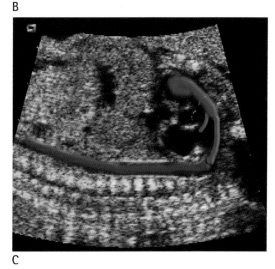

C

Figure 4.2   **A.** The entire heart seen by superimposition of transparent images. **B.** Complete left outlet. **C.** Complete right outlet.

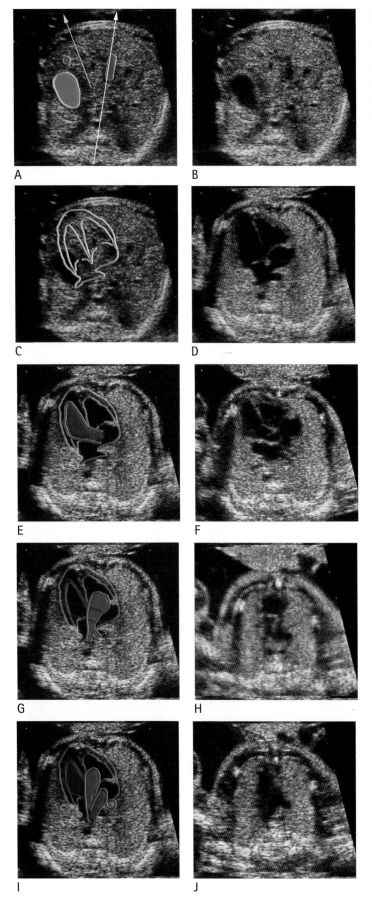

Figure 4.3 Cranial translation from the TAD. **A, B.** Lateralization of the fetus with the stomach; axis of the heart (green arrow). **C, D.** Position of the four chambers related to the TAD. **E, F.** LV–Ao related to the four chambers. **G, H.** RV–PT related to the four chambers. **I, J.** Three-vessel view related to be four chambers (Ao, DA, SVC).

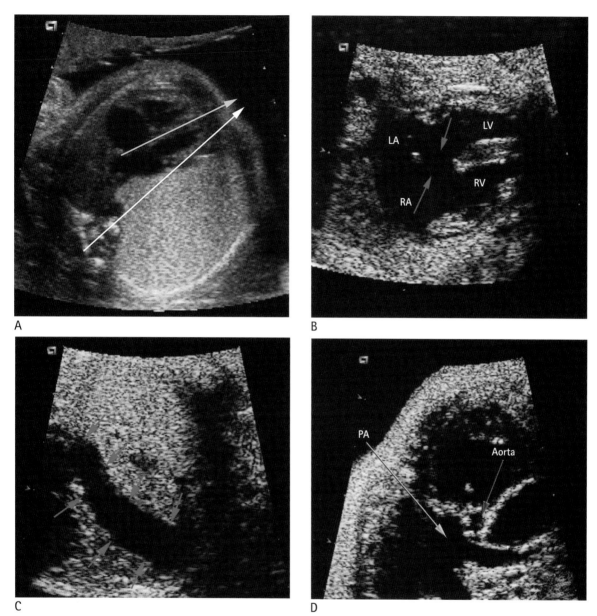

Figure 4.4   These rapid observations allow us to locate certain important features—at least one of these four signs are implicated in most cardiac diseases. **A.** Axial deviation of the heart (green arrow) from the median axis (white arrow) found in situs anomalies, four-chamber asymmetries, and diaphragmatic hernia. **B.** Important defects: aspect of a heart with a large central defect (red arrows) in a complete AVSD. **C.** A great vessel (red arrows) crosses right through the thorax due to an anterior insertion of the aorta, which is a suspicious sign of TGV. **D.** Asymmetries of the great vessels, the outlet. Here, the PA (green arrow) is much greater in size compared to the aorta (red arrow), which implies cardiac anomalies. In a normal situation, the PA is only slightly larger than the aorta.

This rapid observation allows us to locate certain important features such as:

- Situs anomalies.
- Large (volume) defects, e.g. the aspect of a heart which has a large central hole points to a complete atrioventricular septal defect (AVSD).
- The great vessel crossing directly through the thorax with bifurcation, which testifies to an anterior insertion of the aorta leading us immediately to suspect transposition of the great vessels (TGV).
- The outlet and diameter of the great vessels, if abnormal, will imply cardiac anomalies in most cases.

These swift observations, performed at the very beginning of the examination, will influence what we say to the parents by observing their reactions before directly announcing a problem. Not only will this allow us the time to complete the specific screening required for determining our approach to the findings themselves, observing the reactions of the parents will give us the psychological basis to approach them at the end of the examination. Never make an announcement too early or brutally—take your time.

This dynamic and rapid examination can sometimes, if the technical conditions are favorable, extract those referential views that can demonstrate and affirm the elements we are searching for. The possibility of cineloop allows an easier acquisition of the reference scans.

> Contrary to what we might believe, the real difficulty is not in the actual acquisition of these images, but rather in the choice and identification of the best view which highlights these structures.

The first part of the examination is limited to a simple sweep. New possibilities of acquisition in the 4D mode automatically interpret this sweep to acquire volume. We can thus obtain a view in the three spatial planes, avoiding difficulties linked to the handling of the probe when passing from one view to the next. This volume corresponds to a specific given instant but until recently it was not possible to use this technique for the fetal heart

because the acquisition time was too long (especially for a heart beating at 145 beats per minute). With the arrival of the spatiotemporal image correlation (STIC) technique[2,3] we now have the added information of morphological variations as a function of the cardiac cycle. Increasingly we are seeing in the literature that authors consider this technique sufficient,[2] satisfying the needs of our examination for the screening of the heart itself. Based on the same principle of rapid acquisition, some authors have proposed applying this method to the whole exploration of the fetus.[4] They would use this for "diagnosis at a distance" or for teaching using videoconferencing.[5] Another technique, the "inversion mode",[6,7] provides the possibility of combining different techniques such as STIC, "inversion mode", and "B-flow" imaging.[8]

> We should never forget that a 3D, 4D, STIC, or inversion mode can never mitigate the mediocrity of the initial image.

As mentioned earlier, no matter what the method of acquisition, the real difficulty lies in acquiring a good image and not on the identification of these structures themselves. The quality of the acquisition centers on avoiding the bones: the ribs, the spine, and limbs. Remember if the position of the fetus is not favorable to our examination, temporarily abandon a detailed examination of the heart and the aortic arch, then concentrate on other organs that are, for the moment, more approachable. If the back is to the front, we can examine, for instance, the kidneys or the spine, going back to the heart when it is in a more favorable position for the quality views that we desire.

Different views that verify the 10 key points, their pathways, and their pitfalls

After this fast glance, as a general rule, for each view we choose the most favorable pathway to approach it. In short, we look for a perpendicular approach to the structures we are examining.

With each acquisition we must ask ourselves if the screen is showing us an image that is true or false, whether it is reassuring or a cause for concern. These questions must always be uppermost in our minds during the fetal examination. A precise idea of the potential pitfalls will help us avoid false leads, and possibly save us from making the wrong diagnosis.

In the greater part of fetal anomalies, at least one of these views is pathologic:

- The four-chamber view is not comprehensive if we have not observed the complete movement of the atrioventricular valves.
- The continuity LV–Ao.
- The continuity RV–PT.
- The aortic arch.
- The three-vessel view with the horizontal portion of the arterial duct, the aortic arch, and the transverse view of the superior vena cava (SVC), in 2D and Doppler.

Faced with an anomaly in one of these views, we add, according to the pathology we are looking for, one of the following views:

- The arterial duct view exploring: RV–PT–DA–Ao.
- The IVC–SVC (called bicaval incidence).
- The annular view.
- And eventually other more specific views.

For some practitioners the two views (the four-chamber view and the three-vessel view) may be sufficient in systematic screening, but others still feel we need to add the view that incorporates the LV outlet, without forgetting to study flow in color Doppler (Fig. 4.5).

VERIFICATION OF LATERALIZATION AND ITS PITFALLS: THE ELEVATOR

To be certain of the lateralization of the fetus we must begin by clearly determining the left side of the fetus which varies according to how it presents. This has been described in Chapter 3 (Fig. 4.6).

The technique

In the fetus, the lungs are physiologically empty and the liver is large which causes the base of the heart to be horizontal and found in the same plane as that of the ribs and intercostal spaces.

First we should ensure that we have obtained a good view of the TAD with a centered umbilical vein, including the stomach and, if possible, the two adrenal glands. The position of the stomach will be interpreted as verifying the position of the fetus to ensure that it is definitely on the left. Then we go cranially parallel towards the head, continuing in a parallel movement finally reaching the heart using the aorta and the IVC (in the manner of the cables of an elevator). This cranial translation must rest axially, i.e. perpendicular to the axis of the fetal spine, and not necessarily to an imaginary straight cranial–caudal line. This point is of particular importance when the fetus is flexed.

In this way we ensure that the IVC exists and that the aorta is definitely to the left of the spine, on the same side as the stomach. The IVC is situated in front and on the right of the aorta, deviating towards the front in the cranial translation while still remaining in a median plane. The presence of a great vessel of an identical caliber to that of the aorta, which remains straight and parallel to the aorta, should make us suspicious of an azygos vein, and consequently look for the absence of the IVC. This is one of the easiest signs to detect of an important pathology which we will look at later: visceroatrial heterotaxia.

The movement of this caudal translation leads us to the view of a rib and the intercostal spaces which is that of the "optimal" four-chamber view. We have defined this view by the alignment of the apex of the heart and the two inferior pulmonary veins (PVs), a reference point for the four-chamber view.

Pitfalls

The position of the fetus: lateralization elements

These considerations are generally thought to be obvious, but are perhaps more difficult when the fetus is found to be in a transverse position. The fetus might also have moved between the stage of lateralization and that of the examination of the heart.

Organ position

It can be dangerous to be satisfied simply by observing that the stomach is on the same side as the heart.

Normally the stomach is to the left, while the gall bladder is to the right. But what is to the right passes to the left (for the same back position) de-

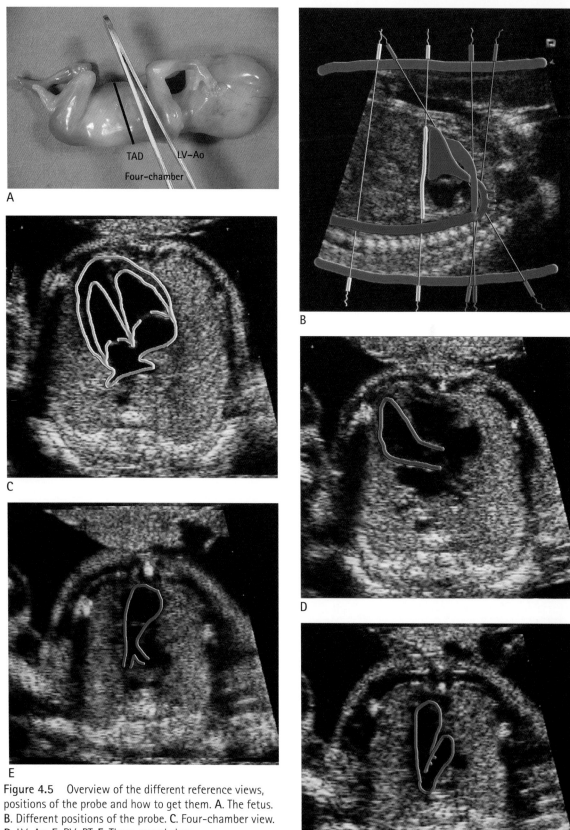

Figure 4.5 Overview of the different reference views, positions of the probe and how to get them. A. The fetus. B. Different positions of the probe. C. Four-chamber view. D. LV–Ao. E. RV–PT. F. Three-vessel view.

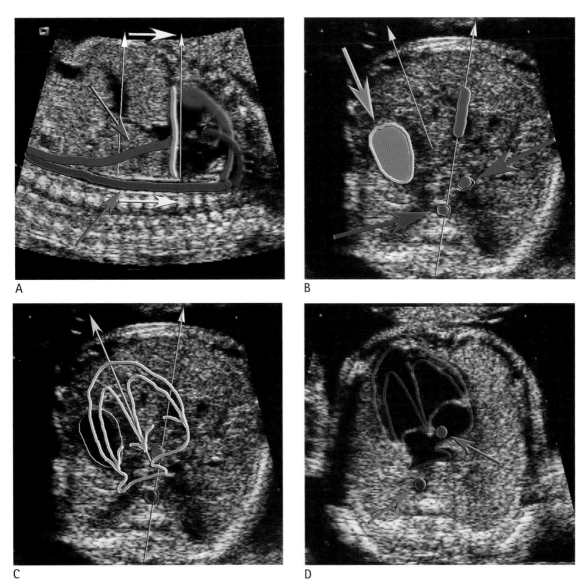

Figure 4.6   **A.** Sagittal view demonstrating the technique of the elevator—parallel movements of the probe from the TAD to the four-chamber view (yellow arrows)—guided using the aorta (red arrow) and the IVC (blue arrow). **B.** TAD; with the stomach (green arrow) we can determine the position and lateralization of the fetus. Using the red and blue lines as guides, we rise to the four-chamber view. Aorta (red arrow) and IVC (blue arrow). **C.** Four-chamber view showing the arrival of the IVC (green arrow) into the right atrium and the aorta behind the left atrium. **D.** Arrival of the elevator compared with the four-chamber view: IVC in the RA (blue point) and the aorta behind the LA (red point).

pending on whether the presentation of the fetus is cephalic or breech. The position of the stomach should be understood as verifying this presentation, i.e. in relation to the position of the head and not of the heart. Forgetting to do this can make us mistake a stomach that is to the right with a gall bladder that is actually to the left.

Abdominal vessel position

It is important to remember to verify that the aorta is truly to the left and that the IVC is present, and comes out into the RA. It is also extremely useful to use the aorta and the IVC as our guides for the "elevator" between the TAD and the four-chamber view. To do this we must search for them, knowing that we will always find the aorta to the left of the spine, and the IVC on the right side of the TAD view of a normal fetus.

A vessel remaining close to the aorta without separating towards the front during a cranial translation—and which has an appearance similar to the barrel of a rifle—should not be taken to be the IVC. It is most probably a voluminous azygous venous return which is confirmed by the absence of a normal image of a vessel in front and on the right of the aorta, the IVC. These elements are easily seen in the TAD view, and also on the parasagittal view of the aortic arch, as long as the fetus is in a neutral position.

Four–chamber view: verification of the outlet and its pitfalls

The technique

As described earlier, examination of this view is obtained from the TAD view, after having gone up in parallel until reaching the heart, the "elevator" guided by the Ao and IVC (Fig. 4.7). Like this we have a four-chamber view (see Figs 4.7H–J) which is "optimally" aligned with these three reference points and the following structures:

- The apex of the heart.
- The two inferior pulmonary veins.
- The ideal level for examining the crux of the heart, and the insertion of the atrioventricular valves.

Due to the position of the fetal heart (empty lungs and large liver), this view is on the same plane as that of the ribs and the intercostal spaces.

> One rib in front and one in the back are excellent criteria in obtaining the optimal four-chamber reference scan (see Figs 4.7H–J; see also Fig. 4.10).

!!! ATTENTION !!!

> It becomes impossible to obtain the three reference points by a parallel translation if the spinal curvature of the fetus is important. In this case, the incidences of the TAD and the four-chamber view are not strictly parallel.
>
> In fact, the movement has to follow the curvature of the spine and remain always perpendicular to it. The movement won't be a parallel translation at all, but a curved movement in the same way that the spine of the fetus itself is curved.

> In every case the cranial translation from the TAD should remain axial, i.e. perpendicular to the axis of the fetal spine and not that of the probe.

If the four-chamber view is not strictly axial, it will be impossible to find the three reference points, but we can also experience pitfalls due to the wrong swing, as shown in Figure 4.8. For instance, in this particular situation it happens when we pass along the apex and the superior—and not the inferior—PVs.

To correct our views, we have a tendency of pivoting the probe around a fixed point on the surface of the skin. What in fact should be done is to move the probe *along* the skin, keeping as a fixed point a chosen interior reference of the view which thus serves as our axis of rotation (Fig. 4.7c).

The choice of different access pathways for the four-chamber view will at first be determined by the position of the fetus and then the pathway. We must make use of three different pathways.

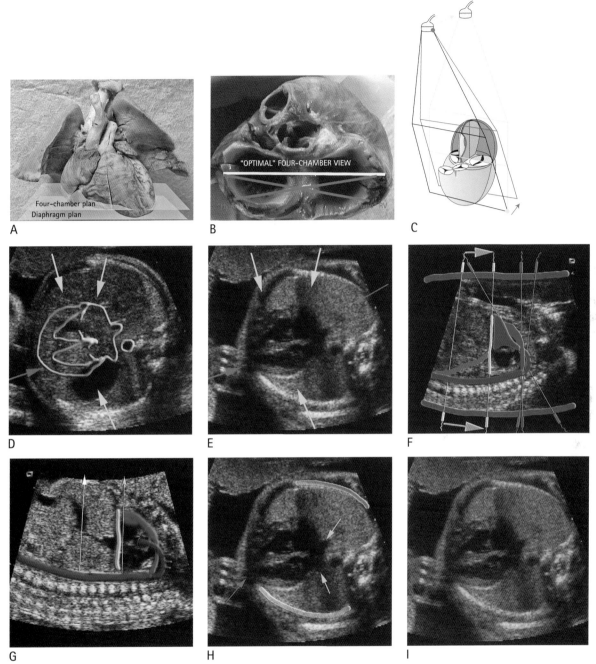

Figure 4.7   **A, B.** Position of the four-chamber view compared with the heart including the pitfalls of this view, a small LV or RV (red lines in "B"). **C.** Going from the red position to the yellow we need to slide the probe on the skin (yellow arrows) turning around the apex (yellow point) and not simply turning the probe without moving it on the skin, as shown on this diagram. (red point). **D.** The position of the fetal organs can be better understood if we superimpose the four-chamber view on the TAD and compare the two. In doing this we can easily determine the best path to take, whether axial–apical (red arrow), axial–transverse (green arrow), or crux of the heart (blue arrow). **E.** The four-chamber view and its pathways. **F.** Here we see the parallelism between the plans of the TAD and the four-chamber view. **G.** Position of the probe in a sagittal view. We can visualize the consequences of the loss of parallelism due to the curved back of the fetus. **H.** Definition of the three points that confirm the four-chamber view. On the same image we have the apex (red arrow) and the two pulmonary veins (blues arrows), with an entire rib (yellow). **I.** Same view as in 'H' but unmarked.

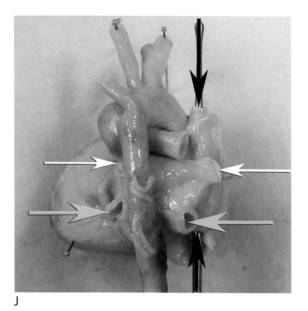
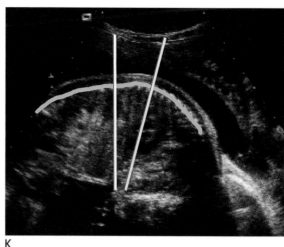

J K

Figure 4.7 (*cont'd*) **J.** Posterior view of PVs: inferior (blue arrows) and superior (white arrows). This view explains the importance of the inferior PVs. Visualization to get an axial view and why they are one of the criteria for the four-chamber view to avoid lateral or anteroposterior swing. **K.** The curved spine lost the parallelism between the TAD (white line) and the four-chamber view (yellow line).

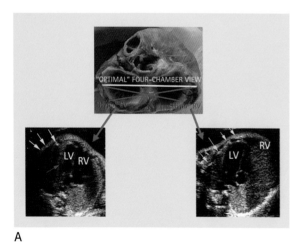
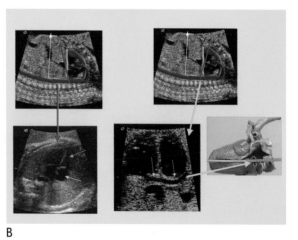

A B

Figure 4.8 **A.** These views demonstrate how a lateral swing can produce false small ventricles (RV or LV) shown with red arrows. Yellow arrows indicate several ribs instead of the usual one in axial views. **B.** Anteroposterior swing. Small ventricles (red arrow) or false AVSD seen in the case of a dilated CS (green arrow).

The axial–apical pathway

This is shown in Figure 4.9.

Why

This is the preferred pathway in pediatric cardiology. Free of any bone obstacles, it is usually easy to obtain in a fetus with a posteriorly positioned back. We can also use this with a fetus with an anterior back by passing by the paraspinal window. This is often possible with a transverse view as early as the first trimester. Especially useful in cases of a bad echogenicity it allows us, by its perpendicular approach, to visualize the closed atrioventricular valves demonstrating their symmetry and offsetting.

How

It is obtained by a cranial translation beginning with the TAD, perpendicular to the axis of the spine with a slight angulation.

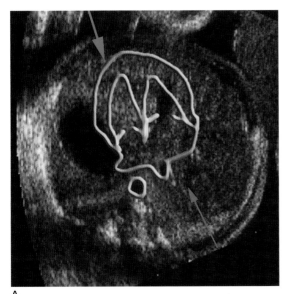

A

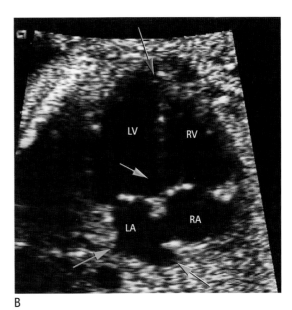

B

Figure 4.9   **A.** Position of the four-chamber view superimposed on the TAD. **B.** Four-chamber view by the apex with the criteria for a reference view: the apex (red arrow) and inferior PVs (blue arrows). With this incidence the limits of the septum are not well defined (green arrow). **C.** The same view with the valves open.

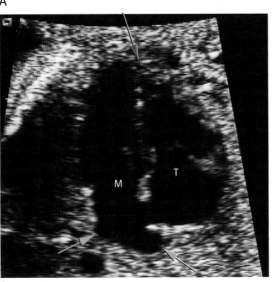

C

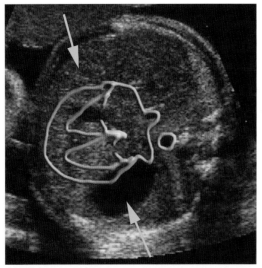

A

Figure 4.10   **A.** The lateral pathway (green arrows) showing the four-chamber view on the TAD by superimposition. **B.** Despite an insufficient zoom this incidence allows us to better visualize the septum. **C.** A correct zoom emphasizes the good visualization of the endocardium (green arrows) because of its perpendicular incidence.

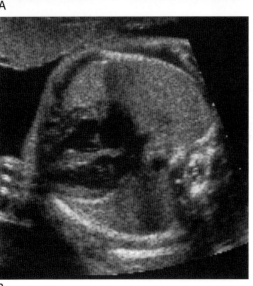

B

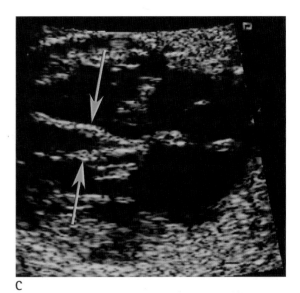

C

!!! ATTENTION !!!

The longitudinal approach to the muscle fibers of the interventricular septum (IVS) generates tangential shadow cones which make it appear thinner than it really is. This can also get in the way of apical visualization of the crux of the heart.

The apical view is never used in measuring the IVS for diabetic pregnancies.

The axial–transverse pathway

This is shown in Figure 4.10.

Why

This approach, often obscured by the ribs, makes viewing the walls easier, especially those of the IVS. Indispensable in measuring the IVS in the diabetic, it is equally of great interest in the study of a complete AVSD where the IVS appears short and squat (Fig. 4.11).

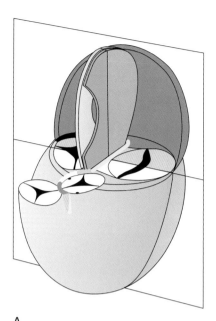

A

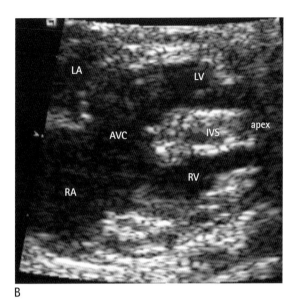

B

Figure 4.11   A. Diagram of the four-chamber view with the valves and their situations. **B.** A large central defect is a sign of an AVSD. **C.** This diagram shows the modifications which occur causing the septum to be large and stubby.

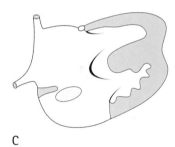

C

View of the crux of the heart

This is shown in Figure 4.12.

Why

This appearance allows us to emphasize the offsetting of the septal atrioventricular leaflets by underlining the obliquity of the fibers linking these valves in their intraseptal section.

How

We must approach the fibers perpendicularly by using the zoom; in this way the fibrous portion (non-muscular), which is normally oblique in relation to the IVS (muscular), appears very echogenic and well-differentiated from the muscle tissue. To emphasize the difference of echogenicity a very high contrast setting can be used.

To be absolutely clear, the study of the offsetting of the atrioventricular valves can only be performed using the "optimal" four-chamber view, i.e. the view defined by the apex and the two inferior PVs.

We understand the heart as having two parts: inlet and outlet. The part concerning inlet corresponds to the four-chamber view.

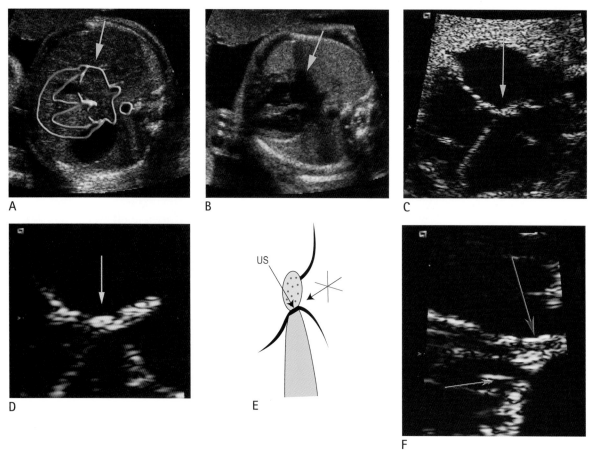

Figure 4.12   A, B. This preferred approach allows a perpendicular approach to the fibers that cross the septum creating a hyperechogenicity due to the mirror effect (blue arrow). C, D. The correct zoom improves our ability to identify hyperechogenic fibers. The greater the zoom, the easier it is to differentiate the fibers of the myocardium. This depends on optimum settings. D–F. Demonstration of the importance of the choice of US angle (white arrow). When it is perpendicular the intramyocardial fibers are hyperechogenic, instead of those in "E" and "F" where the US is not perpendicular (red arrow); this portion of the fibers is ignored. Very echogenic in "D", when the angle of indicence is changed in "F" the fibers become anechogenic. Note the usefulness of a large zoom in better visualizing interseptal fibers.

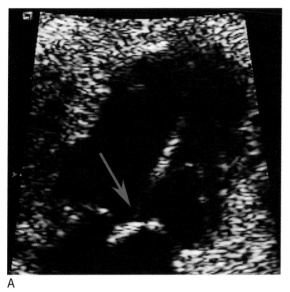
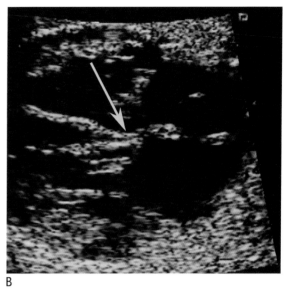

A   B

Figure 4.13   A. Although specific settings can reassure us about the offsetting of the valves, these settings can lead to false images of a defect (red arrow). **B.** In case of doubt it is necessary to change the incidence to be perpendicular showing the septum as normal (green arrow). Notice that by modifying the angle parallel, the fibers are hyperechogenic and seem to "disappear".

!!! ATTENTION !!!

The offsetting of the valves may appear difficult to highlight if access to the fibers has not been accomplished in a perpendicular fashion.

The reason for using a hard-contrast setting is to emphasize the difference between the myocardium and the fibers in continuation with the two atrioventricular valves crossing the septum. This setting can lead to not being able to recognize part of the septum, but this problem can be avoided by changing the trajectory (Fig. 4.13).

and to the left where we find the left atrium in front and to the left of the spine. In conotruncal cardiopathy (CTC) the arch can be to the right, most often going off with a descending aorta to the right as well. This marker—which is very easy to see and is an element of our key points—is a powerful warning sign of a fetal pathology.

The axis of the heart

Normally situated between 30° and 60°, the axis is generally seen to fall around 45°. Values found at either limit should make us suspicious of an asymmetry and lead us to consider an inlet pathology. If the angle is less than 30° it is most likely a hypoplasia of the right ventricle. If the angle is more than 60° it suggests a left hypoplasia.

Pitfalls of the inlet or four-chamber view

The axis of the heart and the aorta to the left

The lateralization of the heart should be noted in relation to the fetal position, not simply in relation to the abdominal organs. The position of the aorta at the level of the four-chamber view is in the back

!!! ATTENTION !!!

The "boot" form—well-described in tetralogy of Fallot—also causes a deviation of the axis to the left.

Swings in the four-chamber view

The axis of the four-chamber view is confirmed by visualization of a whole rib; the optimal level of this view is ensured by visualization in the same plane as the apex of the heart and the inferior PVs. The absence of these criteria is due to a swing, which could be lateral or anteroposterior.

Lateral swings: asymmetries

Lateral swings create false asymmetries either to the right or to the left due to the direction of the swing, whether it is to the left or right (Fig. 4.14).

This view gives the impression of a right or left ventricular hypoplasia. The diagnosis needs to be reconsidered using our criteria to verify the horizontal nature of the view. On these images we cannot see one single complete rib but several. Continuing with the examination, a balanced outlet tract was seen, which would be illogical if a right or left hypoplasia actually existed.

For an inferior–superior swing: false AVSD and VSD

By the same mechanism, if the view is too caudal towards the front, the ventricles will be visualized by

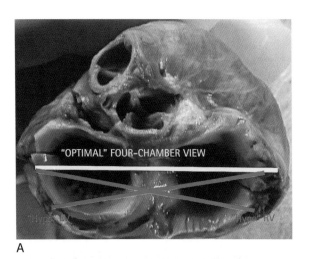

A

Figure 4.14   A. A optimal four-chamber view (yellow line). The lateral swings are shown by a red line. Notice that there are several cut ribs (yellow arrows) in this view, but in the wrong position. B. Angled towards the left, the LV appears falsely small. C. Angled towards the right, the RV appears falsely small.

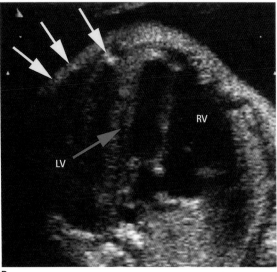

B

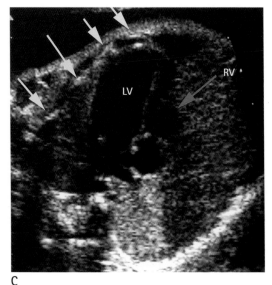

C

their walls and not their chambers (Fig. 4.15A–C). This can increase our impression of hypoplasia if the view also has a lateral swing.

A view which is too caudal towards the back can present us with the following:

- When there is a right swing, we have distracting images such as the visualization of the Eustachian valve situated at the entry of the IVC. Of variable size, it can be seen on one view, even when situated at a good level. Another distracting image in the RA is the presence of Chiari's network, an embryological remnant floating in the RA (Fig. 4.16).
- When there is a left swing you can be confused by the following images.

The CS, especially if it is dilated by the arrival of a persistent LSVC receiving an abnormal pulmonary venous return, easily gives us a false image of the alignment of the atrioventricular valves, implying the existence of an AVSD. If the static image is disconcerting, dynamically we see that these "linear valves" are without any movement because in fact it is the wall of the coronary sinus. In addition, the absence of the arrival of the PVs in a small left atrium should be a warning of this pitfall and lead us to reconsider the level of this four-chamber view—as the absence of a complete rib (Fig. 4.15C, D).

A dilated CS can also be an obstacle to left flow leading us to consider a diagnosis of left hypoplasia or coarctation. Even a normal CS can be visualized on the axial plan of the four-chamber view if this plane is too low. Here as well, the PVs will not be seen arriving in the LA because they come out above the plane of this image. Looking for the ribs will allow us to confirm the absence of even one complete rib confirming the axiality.

On these two images, the presence of several ribs proves that the image has been taken obliquely. This puts in doubt a diagnosis of asymmetry, especially since the axis of the heart is normal, the opposite of a true asymmetry.

When the swing is towards the top, it is not the crux of the heart, but the membranous septum and the base of the aorta which are in the view, easily creating false images of VSD.

These pitfalls can be avoided if we respect the three reference points of the "optimal" four-chamber view, confirmed by seeing: a complete rib; the apex, and the two inferior PVs.

To avoid these pitfalls, we have a tendency to pivot the probe around a fixed point made of skin. On the contrary, it is indispensable to move the probe on the skin while keeping as a fixed point the references of the view which will serve as an axis of rotation; in this case the apex can be used to align the two inferior PVs and reach our three points (Fig. 4.17).

Four-chamber view and concordance

One of the steps in the examination using the four-chamber view is the identification of each of the chambers, which will permit us to judge whether they are concordant or not. The LV has a smooth wall whose apical extremity constitutes the apex of the heart. If there is one left atrium characterized by the arrival of the PVs and then followed by a type of straight ventricle, that is to say having coarse trabeculations, we speak of an atrioventricular discordance. You must pay particular attention to the atrioventricular concordance to be sure not to overlook a double discordance (also called "corrected transposition").

Aspect of a false echogenic tumor of the right ventricle

The apical approach can give us a very echogenic, bulky, and filled image of the back of the RV. This is due to the trabeculations formed by the numerous bridge-like fibers. These fibers give us a multitude of interfaces which are at the origin of the echogenicity that makes this such a distracting image. Color Doppler (ideally used in an apical path) allows us to immediately disprove the presence of a tumor by the total filling of the ventricle. This is accomplished through the visualization, in color Doppler, of blood passing between the muscular bridges and the trabeculations. Moreover, if this happens to be filling defect linked to a hypoplasia or a ventricle tumor, there will be a dilatation upstream with a valvular leak associated with hypoplasia downstream, that is to say of the pulmonary artery (Fig. 4.18).

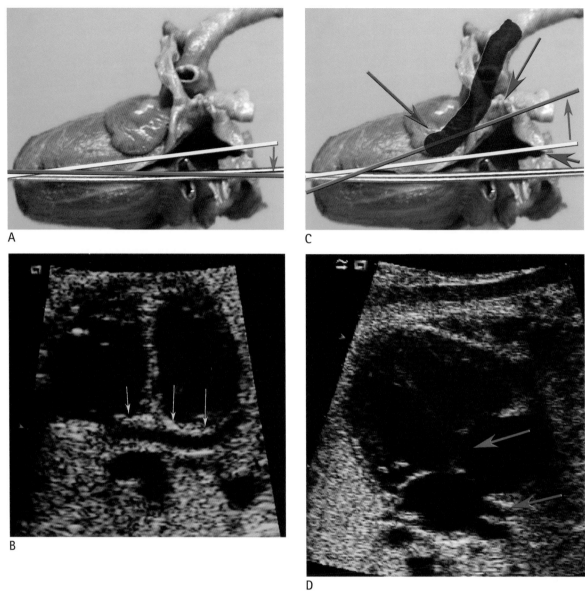

Figure 4.15   The four-chamber reference view is illustrated by a yellow line. **A.** Anatomic view. An inferior swing (red arrow) uncovers the CS in such a way that it can be mistaken for an AVSD. **B.** This section of the dilated CS gives a false image of AVSD, which disappears when we perform a cranial translation to look at the integral crux of the heart. Note that this CS can be dilated, especially if it receives a persistent SVC. **C.** If there is an upward swing (red arrow), the four-chamber view elucidates the superior PVs and the beginning of the aorta. This view, which passes by the superior PVs and by the inferior portion of the beginning of the of the aorta, gives a false image of a VSD—a septal defect which is too cephalic and anterior. **D.** Sonographic correspondence with the departure of the aorta creates a false image of a defect (red arrow) as the PV visualized is the superior one (blue arrow) not the inferior.

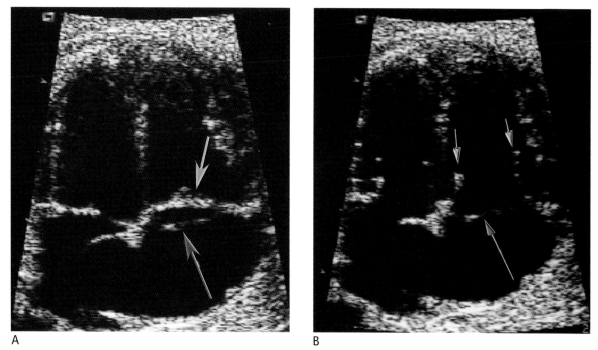

Figure 4.16   A. A double echogenic line due to the tricuspid (green arrow) and Chiari's network (red arrow). B. When the tricuspid is open, there is persistence of the echogenic line of Chiari's network.

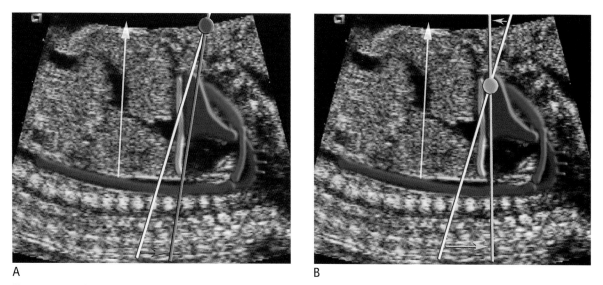

Figure 4.17   A. To obtain the four-chamber view, using the skin as an axis of rotation (red point) makes it impossible to get an optimal reference scan. B. On the other hand, one reference point (here the apex is shown as a green point) is an excellent axis of rotation (green point) to obtain the optimal four-chamber view.

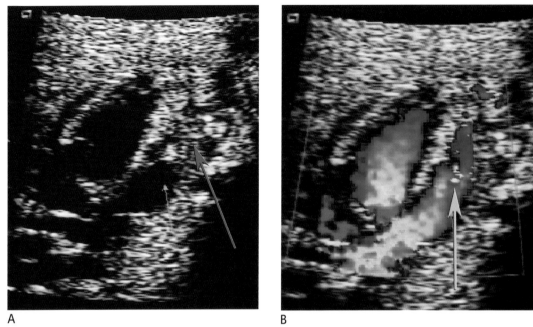

A   B

Figure 4.18   A. Hyperechoic structures occupying all the back of the right ventricular cavity (red arrow). B. The flow in color mode completely fills the ventricle (green arrow), which rules out the possibility of a ventricular tumor. It is simply the tight chordae that result in numerous interfaces.

Four-chamber view and foramen ovale valve

Beware of the pitfalls that involve the foramen ovale valve (FOV) and the LA. In the most severe hypoplasias of the left tracts, or if a left obstacle is important, an authentic FOV can be found in the right atrium. But we should be cautious because the Eustachian valve which sits over the arrival of the IVC could be confused in certain rare cases with the FOV. This valve can be identified especially when the four-chamber view is relatively low and/or the Eustachian valve is particularly large.

The FOV can also sometimes be seen to have an aneurism forming a sac looking like a spinnaker.

Verification of the outlet and its pitfall

The LV–Ao view

The aorta begins at the center of the heart above the inlet and under and behind the PT. Its ascending trajectory is followed by an arch which gives off the vessels of the neck before rejoining the descending Ao (Fig. 4.19).

The technique

The LV–Ao view is obtained from the four-chamber views by a rocking movement of the probe with the apex for the axis. This can be compared to the opening of a "book". The angulation of this four-chamber view, LV–Ao, is about 15°. It is in this zone that we find the membranous septum (MS), at the junction of the inlet and outlet. As in the four-chamber view, the close passage of the LV–Ao view to the MS should be avoided. This would indicate that the level is too caudal, the thinness of the MS easily producing a false image of a defect. It is thus important to produce an LV–Ao view at the level where the septal–aortic continuity is fibromuscular, i.e. more cranial.

There are three important principal pathways, as follows.

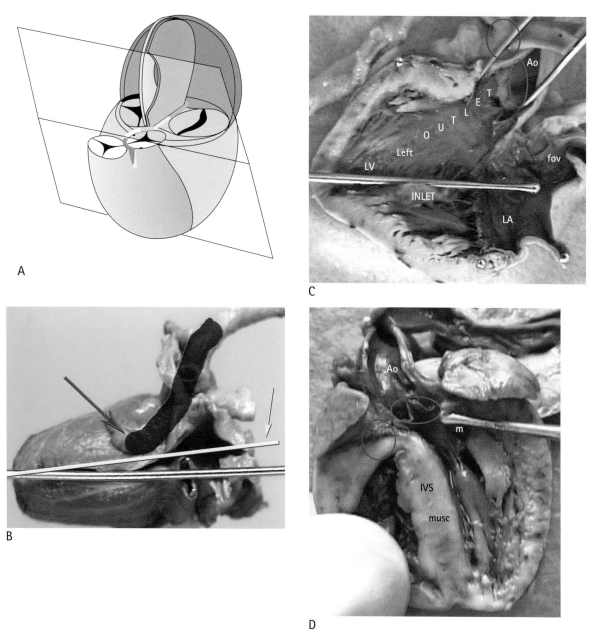

Figure 4.19 **A.** Diagram of the left outlet. Note the acute angle made with this and the four-chamber view. **B.** The origin of the aorta is at the center of the heart (red arrow), close to the plane of the four-chamber view (yellow arrow). **C, D.** Lateral view of the septum from the LV. Anatomic demonstration of the origin of the aorta, close to the center of the heart (red ring) as compared to the right tract, which is more anterior and superior (blue ring).

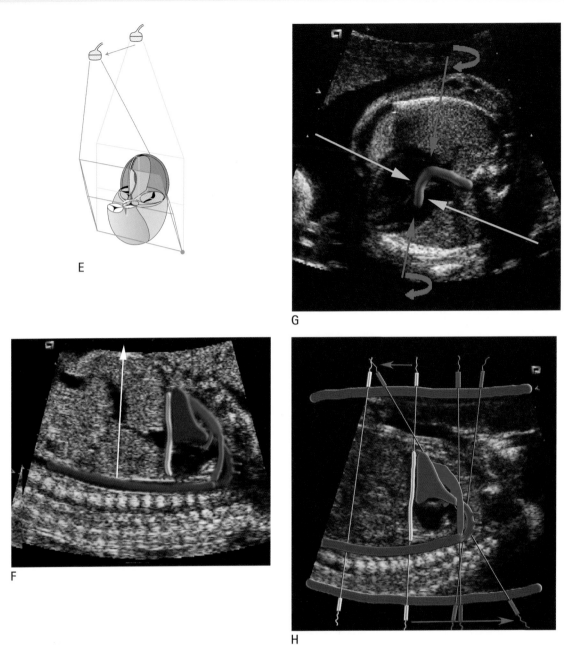

Figure 4.19 (cont'd) E. Description of the movement to go from the four-chamber view to the left-outlet view. It seems natural to angle the probe, keeping it at the same place on the skin. In fact doing this makes reaching this frame impossible, as explained in this diagram, because the center of rotation of this movement must use the apex and not the skin. Otherwise, the probe has to move over quite an expanse of skin. F. Surrounding the left outlet. G. Different pathways as a function of fetal position. Axial–apical (red arrows), axial–lateral (green arrows), and sagittal–oblique (red curved arrows: rotation on the axis represented by the straight arrows). E, H. How to get an axial view of the left track.

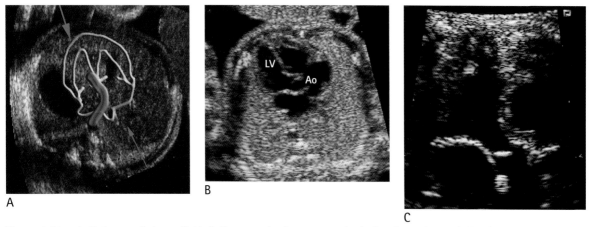

Figure 4.20   **A.** Pathways. **B.** Large field. **C.** The zoom is always a good solution for easier analysis of the structures.

The axial–apical LV–Ao view

This is shown in Figure 4.20.

Why

This is easy to obtain in the continuity of the apical four-chamber view. It is used, above all, in the case where the positioning of the back is posterior.

If there remain any doubts, the use of color Doppler is especially efficient if the US beam is in the same axis as the supposed flow (Fig. 4.21).

The systematic use of color Doppler can also allow the highlighting of small aortic valvular irregularities leading us to look for evidence of a bicuspid condition (Fig. 4.22).

> **!!! ATTENTION !!!**
>
> This view can generate cones of shadow, in particular at the emergence of the aorta, which can suggest a VSD with misalignment. In order to verify the integrity of the septum, it is better to change the incidence angle and approach perpendicularly.

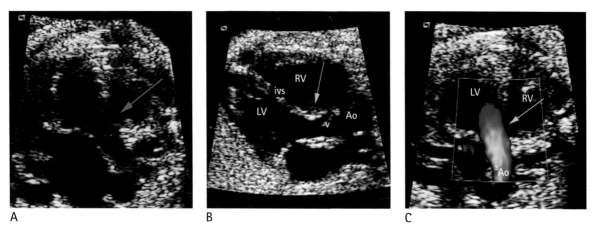

Figure 4.21   **A.** There is some doubt about this septum (red arrow) due to the absence of echoes at this location. **B.** Changing incidence angle often resolves this doubt (green arrow). **C.** Use of color Doppler confirms that the aorta does not receive any flow from the right track at its origin. We can be sure of this because the US is perpendicular to the flow.

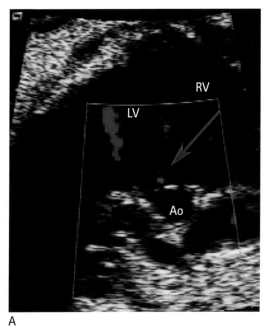

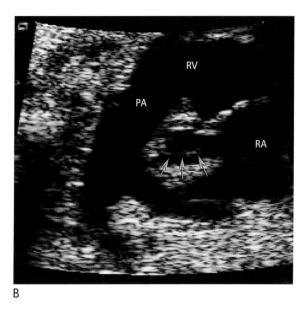

A

Figure 4.22 **A.** Minor regurgitation of the aortic valve. **B.** These data lead us to study the anatomy of the aortic valve more precisely and choose the best pathway to arrive in front of the junction of the valves when they are closed. This echogenic line crosses the valvular anuli demonstrating that there were only two valves instead of three.

The preferred axial–lateral view

This is shown in Figure 4.23.

Why

This view gives the opportunity to explore the outlet VSD. The visualization of the aortic wall is optimal and the approach is perpendicular. It allows us to locate short and thick ventricular septa which are present in the larger defects.

The LV–Ao "SOS" view: sagittal oblique

This view is *only* acquired if the lateral axial approach to the emergence of the aorta is absolutely impossible (Fig. 4.24).

Why

While SOS highlights the infundibular part of the septal–aortic continuity, it leaves certain outlet VSDS untouched especially because it does not explore the wall under the aorta where misalignment defects are situated.

How

As it is impossible to pass from the four-chamber view to an axial or lateral LV–Ao view, we begin by placing ourselves on the LV–RA axis, and then make a 90° rotation. The LV–Ao axis is then approached with a vertical orientation that is slightly oblique (see Fig. 4.22).

Pitfalls of the LV–Ao view

The same problems are encountered with this view as with the four-chamber view (Fig. 4.25). They are due to the incident tangent of the US which can be produced on the LV–Ao view with an approach by the apex. These phenomena will be increased when the axial view is too caudal or where the MS is so thin that it is easy to mistake it for a false VSD. Changing the incidence to arrive perpendicularly into this questionable zone will allow us to find another image of the septum, eventually reduced to an image of interfaces which are composed of the atrioventricular section of the MS. If changing the

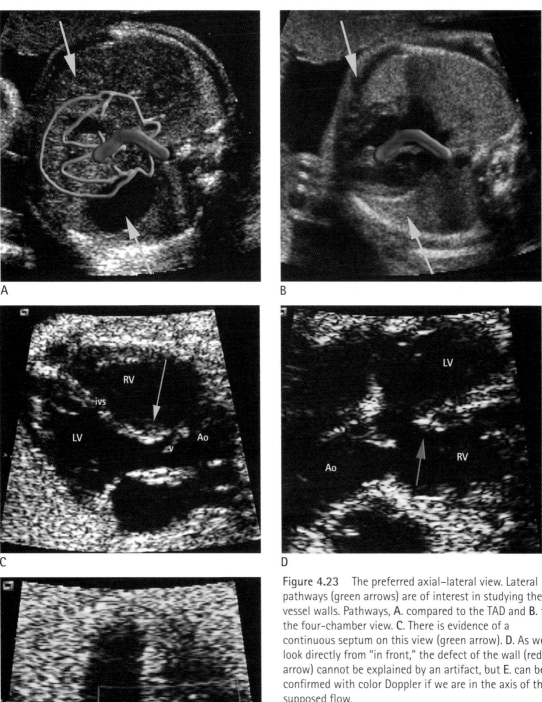

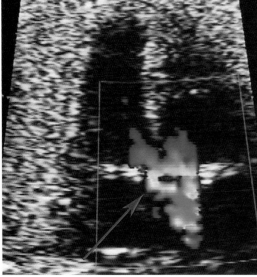

Figure 4.23 The preferred axial–lateral view. Lateral pathways (green arrows) are of interest in studying the vessel walls. Pathways, **A.** compared to the TAD and **B.** to the four-chamber view. **C.** There is evidence of a continuous septum on this view (green arrow). **D.** As we look directly from "in front," the defect of the wall (red arrow) cannot be explained by an artifact, but **E.** can be confirmed with color Doppler if we are in the axis of the supposed flow.

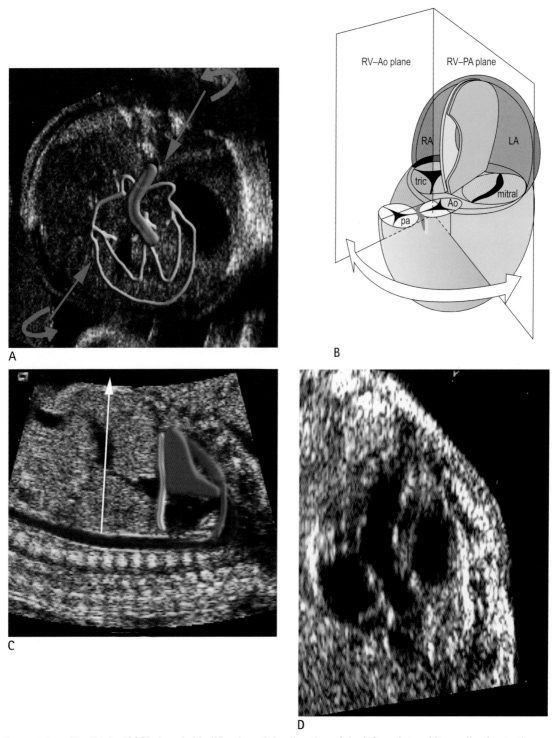

Figure 4.24 The LV–Ao "SOS" view. **A.** Modification of the direction of the left outlet and its application to the pathway for observing the origin of the aorta. **B, C.** Diagrams representing the orthogonal angle between the left outlet as explored by an axial–lateral view and a sagittal view. **D.** Ultrasound perpendicular to the axis of the aorta.

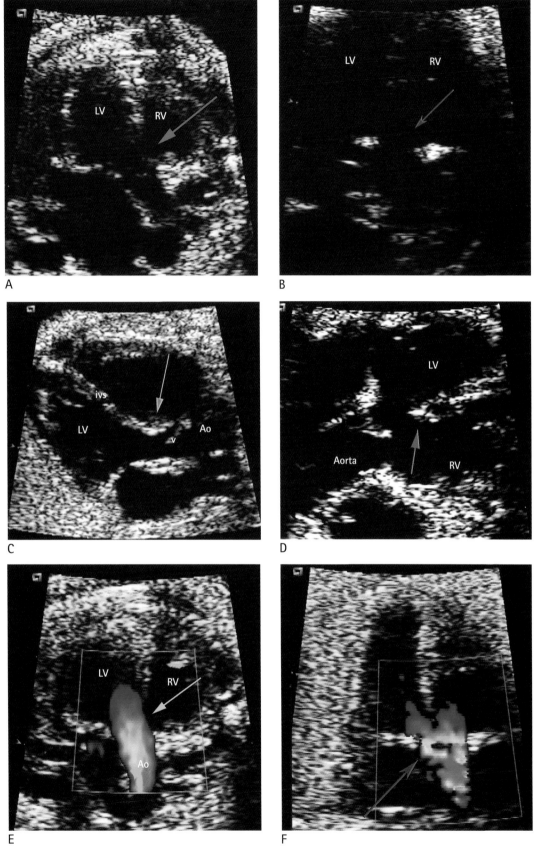

Figure 4.25 Pitfalls of the LV–Ao view. **A.** True VSD. **B.** False VSD. Correcting the pitfall by changing incidence. **C.** No defect (green arrow). **D.** Real defect (red arrow). Doppler provides the diagnosis. Pitfalls of the mLV–Ao view. **E.** No flow coming from the RV (green arrow) in contrast to. **F.** This illustrates where the connection does exist (red arrow).

incidence does not clarify this artifact, we can further sensitize the examination by investigating the flow with color or energy Doppler.

We should note that the sagittal approach to the LV–Ao view—which really deserves its reputation as the "SOS" view when the fetal position limits other approaches—can, at the same time, lead us to mistake a VSD caused by misalignment because this view only examines the wall anterior to the aorta, as well as the infundibular region, but not at all any misalignment under the aorta.

The RV–PT view

The PT, with its practically rectilinear and axial trajectory, arises in the RV in the anterosuperior part of the heart (Fig. 4.26). After having produced the two PAs on its posterior inferior side, where the right artery wraps round the aorta, it continues its straight route by the ductus arteriosus before joining the descending aorta.

Its early bifurcation is the only pathognomonic criteria of the PA (Fig. 4.27).

> A vessel with an early bifurcation is a pulmonary artery. If it comes from the left ventricle it is the very definition of a ventricular arterial discordance, something which is always seen in transposition of the great vessels.

Axial transverse view

This is shown in Figure 4.28.

Why

This view allows us to be perpendicular to the PA wall which, because of the nature of the approach,

appears little echogenic. It is very useful when conditions are difficult.

How

This is ideally from the axial lateral four-chamber view. It is sufficient to effect a cranial translation to make appear a tubular image whose bifurcation rapidly guarantees that this is the PA. A perpendicular view of the PA where the sigmoid valves are shut is preferably chosen as a recorded frame because they generate a small median, which underlines their normal mobility.

View of the right tract, small axis

This view is close to the anatomic view called the ductus arteriosus (DA) (Fig. 4.29).

Why

More complete, yet difficult to produce, it allows us to see all of the right tract with a single view: RA; RV; PT; and DA.

How

Beginning with the four-chamber view, we manage a cranial translation of the probe, by making an oblique movement to the left.

Pitfalls of the RV–PT view

At the level of the great vessels there is a serious risk of confusing the aorta for a PA, creating the false diagnosis of a TGV by mistaking a ventricular arterial discordance.

If we recognize an Ao by three vessels emerging from its arch, it is the early bifurcation of the PA that confirms that we are in effect dealing with the trunk of the PA.

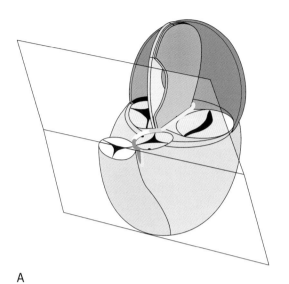

A

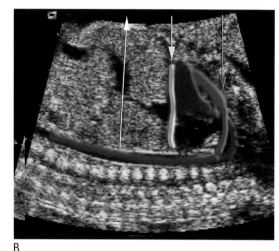

B

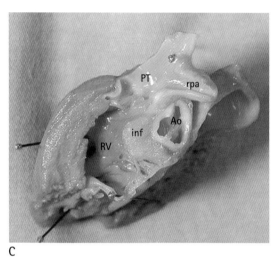

C

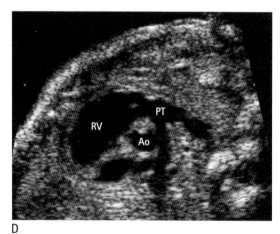

D

Figure 4.26   RV–PT view. A, B. Situation of the axial RV–PT and sagittal RV–PT views as placed in the heart. C. Anatomic and D. US correlations. E. How to get it: as many different pathways as possible. The transverse path (red arrows) is preferable in 2D because it arrives perpendicularly to the PA wall. The axial pathway (green arrows) is preferable in color Doppler because the US is in the direction of flow.

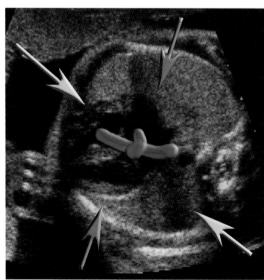

E

The three-vessel view or the two crosses

This is shown in Figure 4.30. This view, first described by Yoo in 1997 and 1999,[9,10] has been quickly developed and its increasing importance, due in part to the simplicity and quickness in obtaining it as compared to the long axis view of the aorta,[11] gives us a summary of more or less all outlet pathologies such as the aortic arch,[12] and often disorders of inlet. Normal values were established for each vessel.[13]

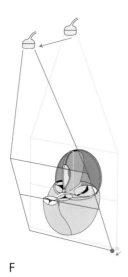

F

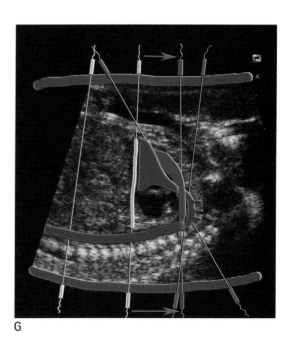

G

Figure 4.26 (*cont'd*)   F, G. Movements of the probe.

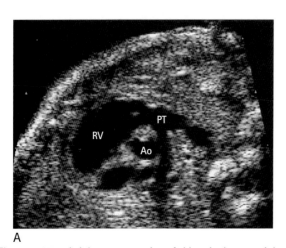

A

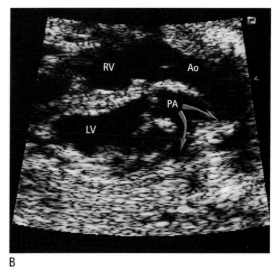

B

Figure 4.27   Axial transverse view. **A.** Ventricular–arterial concordance RV–PT. **B.** Discordance is illustrated by the fact that the vessel with an early bifurcation (red arrows) is a PT coming out of the LV in a TGV.

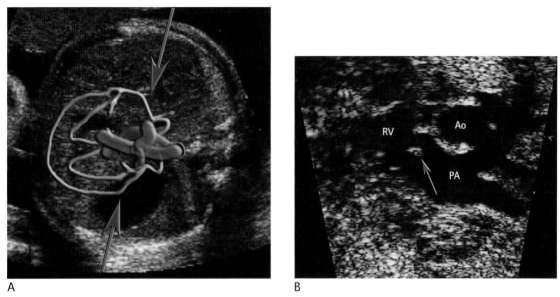

Figure 4.28   **A.** Transverse path perpendicular to the PT wall. **B.** Good echogenicity of the wall. The meeting point of the pulmonary valves (blue arrow) in the center of the vessel confirms the normality of their movements.

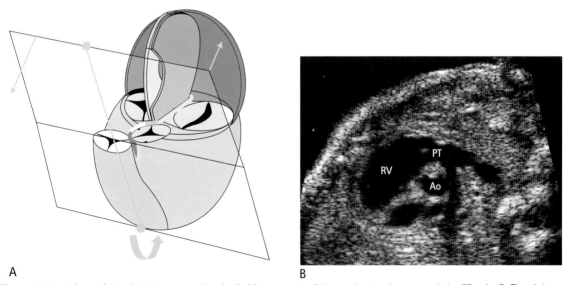

Figure 4.29   View of the right tract, small axis. **A.** Movements of the probe turning around the PT axis. **B.** The right outlet opening is "unrolled."

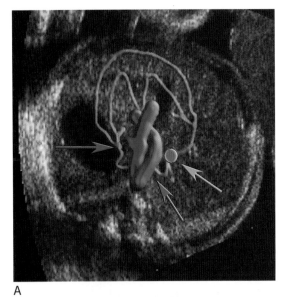

A

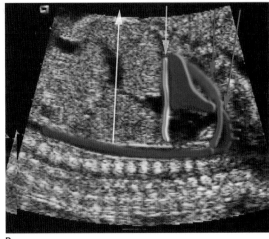

B

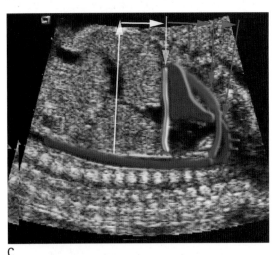

C

Figure 4.30 The three-vessel view or the two crosses. A, B. Situation of the axial and sagittal views as placed in the heart. C. How to get it: parallel translation from the TAD to the three-vessel view, meeting the four-chamber view. This shows a very short left outlet, then the right outlet arising to the three-vessel view. D, E. Anatomic–US correlations.

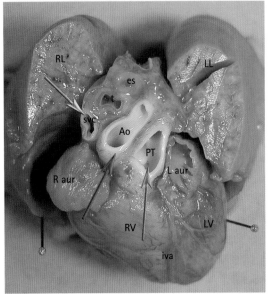

D

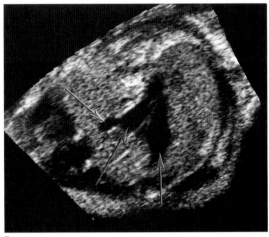

E

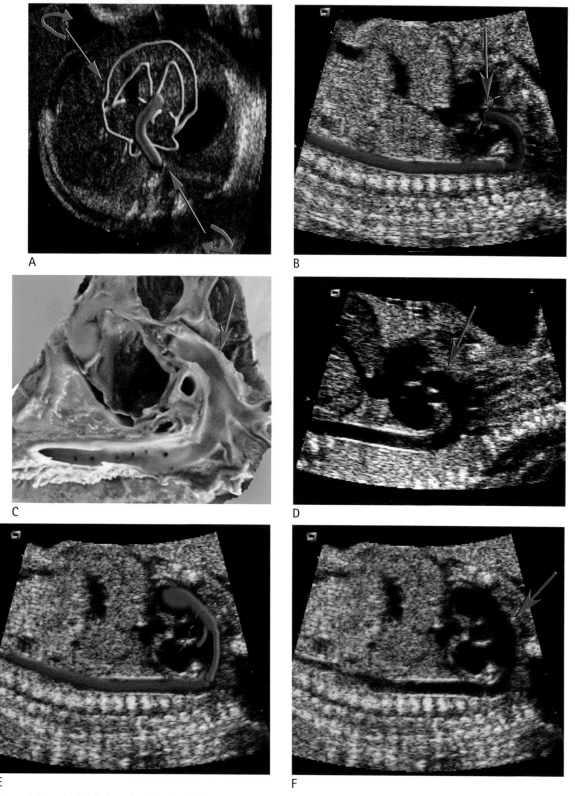

Figure 4.31 **A.** Axial view showing the different directions between the origin of the aorta and the aortic arch (in red) compared with the four-chamber view (in yellow) and the TAD. The aortic arch is viewed starting with an orthogonal translation (curved arrows) from the top of the arch on a three-vessel view. Note the position of the sigmoid valves: pulmonary (small blue arrow) and aortic (small red arrow), more posterior and inferior in the center of the heart. This gives us a narrow hooked cross (large red arrow) that will be enlarged of the aorta receives the RV flow. In this case the origin of the aorta would be at the RV outlet, shown with the large blue arrow. **B–D.** Anatomic correlations. **E–F.** Ductal arch showing its anterior and superior origin (large blue arrow), giving a normal enlarged cross compared to the aortic arch ("B", "F").

Why

This view visualizes, from left to right, the ductal arch, the aortic arch, and then the SVC sectioned transversally. In this way we have reviewed all the outlets of the heart in one single view. Right and left outlet positions are seen and their diameters can be studied, and modified in cases of CTC. It also allows the exploration of the aortic arch, researching interruptions and its posterior diameter, which is particularly interesting in the diagnosis of coarctation at the end of pregnancy. These points were classically researched on the aortic arch sagittal view, but were sometimes very difficult to obtain. The three-vessel view, on the other hand, is almost always possible.

How

This view is, as we have described in the "A fast glance" above, taken in the continuity of the cranial translation: the four-chamber view and RV–PA. By being placed in the axis of the vessels, the use of color Doppler can be a useful complement in difficult cases.

It is wise to finish the examination by color Doppler[14] because verifying that the direction of the flow is in the same direction, as well as the respective speeds of this flow, is a very important element in determining normality.

In paying special attention to the aortic arch (which can already be studied in the three-vessel view in "A fast glance"), any acceleration in flow at the level of the isthmus should suggest the possibility of the formation of a coarctation. The study of flow can be completed by taking the measure in pulsed Doppler just downstream of the origin of the left subclavian artery.

In certain pathologies, it allows us to rapidly identify a retrograde flow, which is a serious element involved in ductal dependence.

Pitfalls of a normal three-vessel view

In reality there are few pitfalls with this view because it allows each outlet structure to be represented in the cardiac outlet architecture so that pathologically at least one of the elements can be seen as "abnormal".

We should not neglect to study flow in the color mode; particularly in the third trimester, reassuring us that we have not picked up any signs of coarctation.

Sagittal view of the aortic arch

This is shown in Figure 4.31.

Why

Verification by this view gives us our a clear "proof positive" of the normal outlet by visualizing:

- The emergence of the aorta in the center of the heart.
- Its regular diameter, without any obvious asymmetry between the anterior and posterior sections of the aortic arch.
- The emergence of the three vessels of the head and neck.

Flow forms the chambers: the diameter and the curve of the arch informs us also of its flow (and indirectly of that of the PA).

Visualization of the complete arch is, outside of this, useful in the diagnosis of pathologies: aortic interruption or coarctations of the aorta.

!!! ATTENTION !!!

The aortic arch should not be confused with that which describes the RV–PT–DA or the ductal arch, for these two axes are only separated by about 10°. The trajectory of the ductal arch is practically axial, but it can be modified due the relative physiologic overload of the right tracts at the end of pregnancy. The ductal arch becomes more rounded and perhaps can be taken then for an aortic arch. Particular attention should be taken of the anterior and superior curve, which is absent in the case of interruption of the aortic arch.

How

The approach of the aorta is achieved in a slightly oblique sagittal plane by the anterior or posterior pathway. This is done using the left paraspinal window. The aortic arch appears in the form of a candy cane. Just as in the characteristic sign of PA with its bifurcation, only the departure of the vessels of the neck can ensure that this is the aorta. It is important to remember that this pathology occurs mainly after birth when the arterial duct closes.

Pitfalls of the aortic arch view

The principal pitfall consists of confusing the aortic arch with the ductal arch. The origins of the aortic arch are posterior and inferior giving it the form of a candy cane, very regular and with a small radius.

Opposite to this, the origin of the ductal arch, more anterior and superior to the PA, leaves it appearing more horizontal.

The aortic arch is identified by the departure of three vessels from the arch.

The confusion, between these two elements can be simplified, especially at the end of pregnancy when the relative overload of the right tract causes it to be elevated, often situated above the aortic arch. If there is the slightest doubt, you should concentrate on showing the existence of the origin of the vessels of the neck, thus identifying the aortic arch.

Only seeing the three vessels exiting from the superior section of the arch can confirm that this is indeed the aorta.

References

1. Sureau C, Henrion R. Rapport du Comité technique de l'échographie de diagnostic prenatal; 2005; www.ladocfrancaise.gouv.fr.
2. De Vore GR, Polanco B, Sklansky MS, Platt LD. The 'spin' technique: a new method for examination of the fetal outflow tracts using three-dimensional ultrasound. Ultrasound Obstet Gynecol 2004; 24(1):72–82.
3. Chaoui R, Hoffmann J, Heling KS. Three-dimensional (3D) and 4D color Doppler fetal echocardiography using spatio-temporal image correlation (STIC). Ultrasound Obstet Gynecol 2004; 23(6):535–545.
4. Benacerraf BR, Shipp TD, Bromley B. How sonographic tomography will change the face of obstetric sonography: a pilot study. J Ultrasound Med 2005; 24(3):371–378.
5. Vinals F, Mandujano L, Vargas G, Giuliano A. Prenatal diagnosis of congenital heart disease using four-dimensional spatio-temporal image correlation (STIC) telemedicine via an Internet link: a pilot study. Ultrasound Obstet Gynecol 2005; 25(1):25–31.
6. Lee W, Goncalves LF, Espinoza J, Romero R. Inversion mode: a new volume analysis tool for 3-dimensional ultrasonography. J Ultrasound Med 2005; 24(2):201–207.
7. Goncalves LF, Espinoza J, Lee W, Mazor M et al. Three- and four-dimensional reconstruction of the aortic and ductal arches using inversion mode: a new rendering algorithm for visualization of fluid-filled anatomical

structures. Ultrasound Obstet Gynecol 2004; 24(6):696–698.
8. Goncalves LF, Espinoza J, Lee W et al. A new approach to fetal echocardiography: digital casts of the fetal cardiac chambers and great vessels for detection of congenital heart disease. J Ultrasound Med 2005; 24(4):415–424.
9. Yoo SJ, Lee YH, Kim ES et al. Three-vessel view of the fetal upper mediastinum: an easy means of detecting abnormalities of the ventricular outflow tracts and great arteries during obstetric screening. Ultrasound Obstet Gynecol 1997 9(3):173–182.
10. Yoo SJ, Lee YH, Cho KS. Abnormal three-vessel view on sonography: a clue to the diagnosis of congenital heart disease in the fetus. Am J Roentgenol 1999; 172(3):825–830.
11. Yagel S, Arbel R, Anteby EY et al. The three vessels and trachea view (3VT) in fetal cardiac scanning. Ultrasound Obstet Gynecol 2002; 20(4):340–345.
12. Achiron R, Rotstein Z, Heggesh J et al. Anomalies of the fetal aortic arch: a novel sonographic approach to in-utero diagnosis. Ultrasound Obstet Gynecol 2002; 20(6):553–557.
13. Zalel Y, Wiener Y, Gamzu R et al. The three-vessel and tracheal view of the fetal heart: an in utero sonographic evaluation. Prenat Diagn 2004; 24(3):174–178.
14. Chaoui R, McEwing R. Three cross-sectional planes for fetal color Doppler echocardiography. Ultrasound Obstet Gynecol 2003; 21(1):81–93.

Further reading

Allan L, Sharland G, Cook A. Fetal cardiology. London: Mosby-Wolfe; 1994.

Batisse A. Cardiologie pédiatrique pratique, 2° édn. Paris: Doin; 2004.

Chaoui R. Fetal echocardiography: state of the art of the state of the heart. Ultrasound Obstet Gynecol 2001; 17(4):277–284.

David N. Echocardiographie fœtale, 2° édn. Paris: Masson; 2002.

Dupuis C, Kachaner J, Freedom RM et al. Cardiologie pédiatrique, 2° édn. Paris: Flammarion; 1991.

Fredouille C. Ultrasonographically normal fetal heart. J Radiol 2000; 81(12):1721–1725. In French.

Ho SY, Baker EJ, Rigby ML, Anderson RH. Congenital heart disease. London: Mosby-Wolfe; 1995.

Larsen WJ, Sherman L. Human embryology, 3rd edition. Edinburgh: Churchill Livingstone; 2001.

Chapter 5

Why: critical cardiac pathologies not to be overlooked

by Catherine Fredouille

 This chapter is also covered in Part 5 of the accompanying DVD

We are now going to describe, in the order they might present, the principle cardiac pathologies that are encountered prenatally.

FIRST STEP. PATHOLOGIES OF POSITION

Pathologies of position are the first we look for when examining the fetal heart. Beginning the examination abdominally, we observe the following.

Anomalies of visceral positioning

In the case where the stomach and heart are not on the same side (Fig. 5.1), the anomaly is clear. More easily overlooked is the case where the stomach is positioned on the right of the fetus along with the heart, a situation which has the same pathologic relevance.

> This implies a systematic verification of the left of the fetus, using the Situs Wheel, not simply checking the homolaterality of the heart and stomach.

Situs anomalies often go unnoticed until the fetal–pathologic or postnatal examinations.[1] They are frequently associated with complex cardiopathies and only worsen the prognosis. These anomalies belong to the visceroatrial heterotaxias (VAH) group with risk of recurrence.

In VAH, gene lateralization anomalies[2] encourage the formation of two homologous sides. Schematically, the fetus that presents with VAH, instead

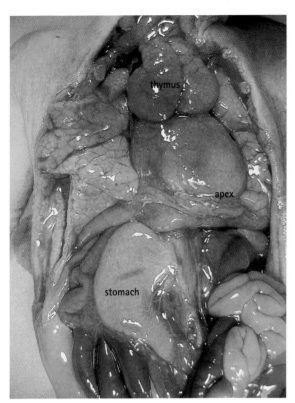

Figure 5.1   The apex of the heart towards the left and the stomach in the right side in a VAH.

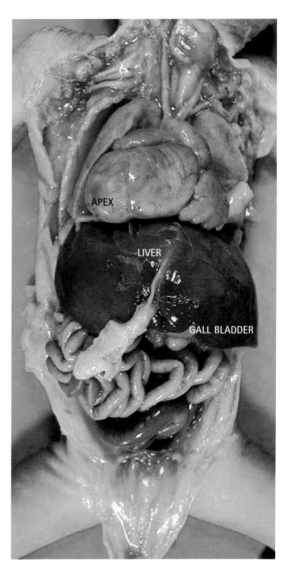

Figure 5.2   Median liver in VAH. Note on the right the apex of the heart, which is not normal.

of having a normal left side and a normal right side has a "doubling," which is neither really left nor right. These abdominal abnormalities are not systematic. They typically affect the liver which becomes median (Fig. 5.2) with the gall bladder situated to the right or left. The spleen, an organ normally found on the left, is classically absent (asplenia) in the case of a right isomerism, or multiple (polysplenia) in the case of a left isomerism. These anomalies are difficult to see with ultrasound (US), especially if we do not systematically verify the lateralization of the vessels and the organs at the abdominal level.

At the same time, prenatally, it is impossible to locate two atrial appendages of the same type which would define a right or left isomerism. But this type of atrial appendage "absence" is often accompanied by anomalies of venous return corresponding to the appendage that is "missing." In left isomerism (two left-type appendages, and therefore no atrium of the right type) the anomaly is found in the systemic venous return which normally would occur in the

"missing" right atrium (RA). This is abnormal and is the reason why we can observe an azygous return (Fig. 5.3) with absence of the suprarenal section of the inferior vena cava (IVC), an element which can be recognized in US[3] by a transverse (Fig. 5.4) or longitudinal (Fig. 5.5) view. In addition, this absence of the RA—which is the normal center for the principal elements of the conduction system—can provoke rhythm problems. In a right isomerism, where the left appendage is missing, we need to consider searching for anomalies related to pulmonary venous return (PVRs), i.e. total or partial PVR.

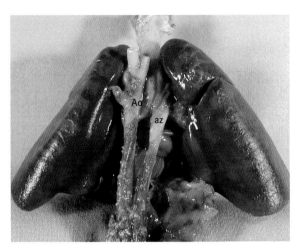

Figure 5.3   Posterior view with a dilated azygos rejoining the superior vena cava (SVC).

These anomalies, even discordant,[4] justify the systematic verification of the abdominal vessels[5] at the level of the transabdominal diameter (TAD), as well as the PVs which attach the heart to the lungs at the level of the four-chamber view.

Vessel position anomalies

In requiring verification of the vessels at the level of the TAD, following them through the "elevator", then arriving at the four-chamber view, we can observe several possibilities.

Not one but two vessels in front and to the left of the spine on the TAD image

These are behind the LA in the four-chamber view (see Figs 5.4 and 5.5). This is the situation in an azygous venous return, classically observed in cases of left isomerism with the absence of a section of the IVC seen at the level of the TAD image.

Though not frequent, and yet of great interest, is the discovery of an infra-diaphragmatic confluent of a totally anomalous PVR (TAPR). When isolated the TAPR can be seen to be recurrent within the same family. This has been observed in the form of a third abdominal vascular mass. It is part of the range of VAH syndromes, and often associated with other pathologic elements of this condition which can be far more difficult to diagnose.

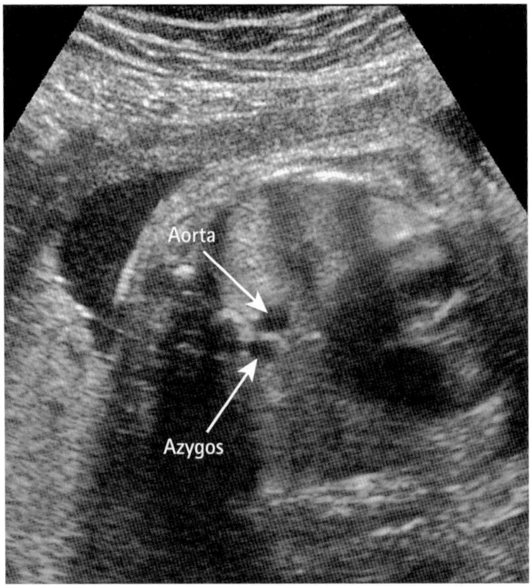

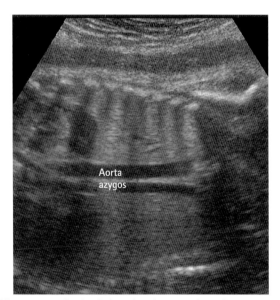

Figure 5.4   Axial US view showing two vessels in front of and to the left of the spine, the aorta, and azygos.

Figure 5.5   Sagittal view showing two thoracic abdominal parallel vessels.

Anomalies of organ or vessel position at the abdominal level, which are present in VAH, are elements of orientation

These are easier to diagnose than the frequent complex CHD associated with them. Often affecting the inlet *and* outlet, VAH cardiopathies found in the inlet are essentially represented by a unique atrium (UA) frequently associated with AVSD or unique ventricle (UV). In the outlet they are often seen as PA with OS, with or without the great vessels being transposed.[6]

To this end, the discovery of an AVSD in a patient having a normal karyotype should immediately lead us to consider VAH.[7]

Visceroatrial heterotaxias present in the form of associations of anomalies of position, inlet, and outlet having a normal karyotype.

The descending aorta is found—not in front and to the left—but on the right of the spine in the four-chamber view

A right descending aorta after a right aortic arch facilitates our diagnosis when we remember to look for it systematically using the four-chamber view. It is an excellent warning sign of conotruncal

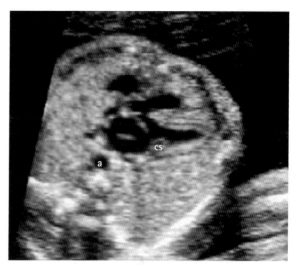

Figure 5.6   "Pediatric" four-chamber view showing a right descending aorta, the axis of the heart (at 60°), and the dilated coronary sinus. We can already see that the VSD predominates in ejection.

cardiopathies (CTC) (Fig. 5.6),[8] the most direct indications for which should only be seen at the outlet level (Fig. 5.7). In addition, this sign, when the standard karyotype is normal, points us towards 22q11 deletion (Fig. 5.8).

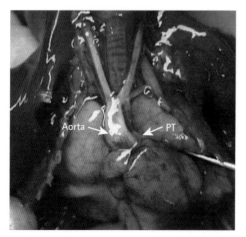

Figure 5.7   Tetralogy of Fallot in trisomy 21 with an arch and right descending aorta. Note the large aorta and the small PT.

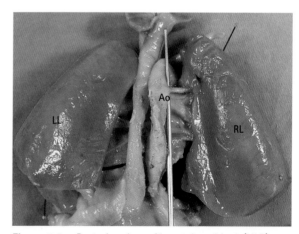

Figure 5.8   Posterior view of heart–lung block (HLB) with the right descending aorta with MAPCA under the probe. This fetus has a 22q11 deletion.

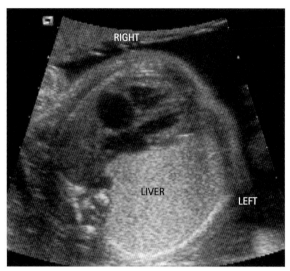

Figure 5.9   Ultrasound view showing the liver in the left hemithorax in a diaphragmatic hernia. The apex of the heart turns towards the left.

Anomalies concerning the position of the heart

The heart is in the right hemithorax (Fig. 5.9), conserving its apex to the left. This case is often associated with a left diaphragmatic hernia (Fig. 5.10). Diaphragmatic hernias are particularly seen in forms of this pathology which are part of a general group of syndromes, (e.g. Fryns syndrome). Associated CHD can also exist here, which would also be generally conotruncal.

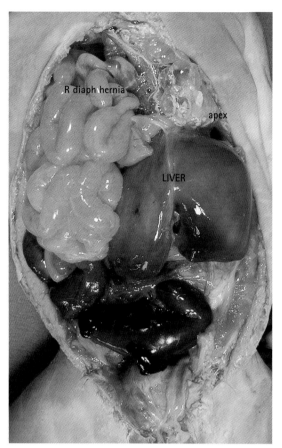

Figure 5.10   Macroscopic view showing liver and intestine in the right hemithorax in a diaphragmatic hernia. The apex of the heart turns towards the left.

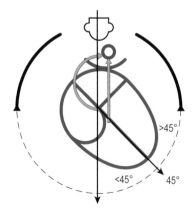

Figure 5.11   Logo of the heart axis.

Anomalies that modify the axis of the heart

The interventricular septum (IVS), which marks the boundary between the right and left inlet tracts, represents the axis of the heart on the four-chamber view. It normally makes a medium-sized angle of 45° with the anteroposterior axis and reflects the balance between the inlet tracts. The right inlet tract is composed of the RA and the inlet section of the RV, while the left inlet tract is composed of the LA and the inlet section of the LV. Any modification of this axis should be observed by the operator during examination using the four-chamber view (Fig. 5.11). Pathologically it is perhaps the asymmetry of the chambers causing an important modification of the axis which attracts our attention.[9]

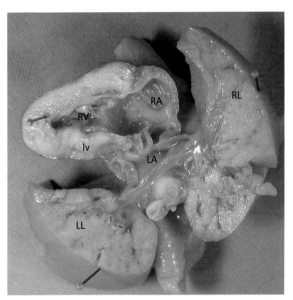

Figure 5.12   Macroscopic view where the axis is at an angle greater than 45° in a hypoplasic LV caused by mitral atresia.

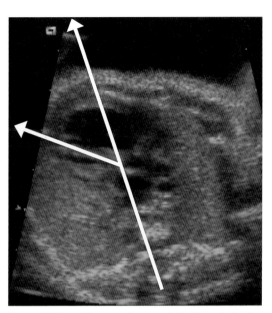

Figure 5.13   Ultrasound view where the axis is at an angle greater than 45° in a hypoplasic LV.

The angle can be clearly superior to 45° with a distinct asymmetry of the chambers

This is seen in severe hypoplasias of the left tracts (Figs 5.12 and 5.13) as well as in Ebstein's disease.

Here (Fig. 5.14) the dilatation of the RA can be enormous due to an incompetent tricuspid valve. This is especially true due to the fact that the septal valve remains stuck to the septum much more than it normally would, enlarging the atrium, which then appears larger than the ventricle. Forms of this anomaly observed prenatally are often severe.

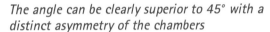

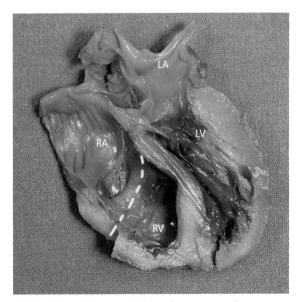

Figure 5.14   Ultrasound view of a macroscopic four-chamber view in Ebstein's disease.

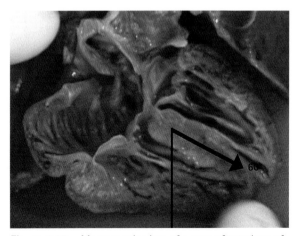

Figure 5.15   Macroscopic view of a case of tetralogy of Fallot with the heart in the classic "boot" shape with an axis of 60°.

The inlet chambers remain symmetric

However, their angle can attain 60° in forms of tetralogy of Fallot (ToF) where the heart takes on the form of a "boot" due to the overriding of the aorta upon the VSD (Fig. 5.15; see also Fig. 5.5).

The angle can be inferior to 45°

This is the case in hypoplasia of the RV called pulmonary atresia with intact septum (PA with IS) (Figs 5.16 and 5.17) that is to say without VSD.[10] Care should be taken not to confuse this condition with pulmonary atresia with open septum (PA with OS), which is a major form of CTC caused by the anterior swing of the conal septum and which has a constant VSD. In the case of PA with IS (exterior to the small size of the PT and RV) fistulae can exist within the coronary circulation on the wall of the RV which are visible on the RV wall in fetal pathology (Fig. 5.18) and translate by multiple aliasing on Doppler. Their hemodynamic consequence can bring about uterine death.[11]

The axis can be negative with the apex of the heart to the right

This could be due to a heart that is a mirror image with complete situs inversus (Fig. 5.19). While cardiac situs inversus is associated with an abdominal situs inversus, this anomaly, which falls in the category of VAH, often remains unnoticed. A dextrorotation due to an atrioventricular discor-dance with a normal atrial situs can also displace the apex towards the right.

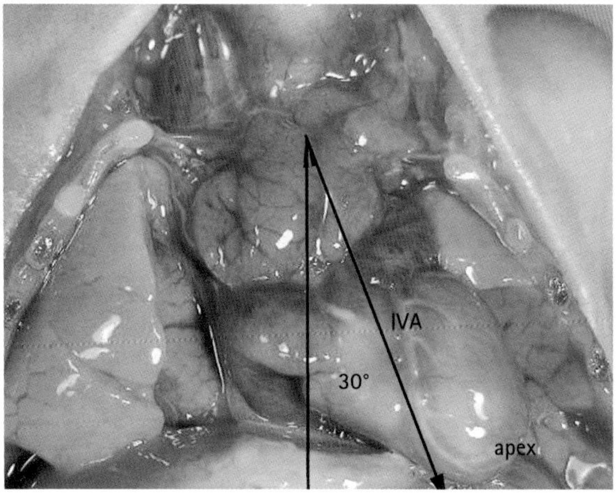

SECOND STEP. PATHOLOGIES OF THE INLET

To each key point, one or several pathologies corresponds:

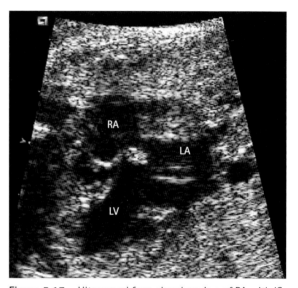

Figure 5.17 Ultrasound four-chamber view of PA with IS.

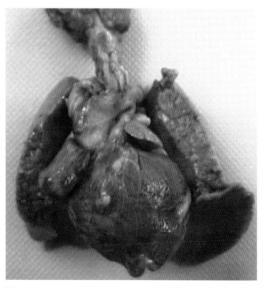

Figure 5.16 Anterior view of the HLB of PA with IS with an axis at an angle less than 45°.

Figure 5.18 Anterior view of the HLB of PA with IS. Note the fistulae.

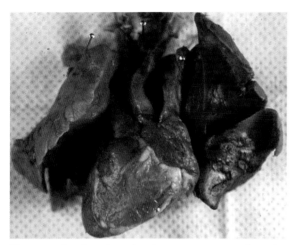

Figure 5.19 Complete situs inversus seen on a thoracic view; the apex of the heart is to the right.

- **Point 3:** heart on the diaphragm, attached by the inferior PV.
- **Point 4:** four chambers.
- **Point 5:** chambers that are balanced and concordant.
- **Point 6:** crux of the heart with permeable and offset rings.

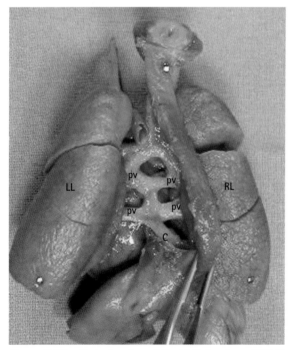

Figure 5.20 Posterior view of the HLB showing a TAPVR with a sub-diaphragmatic confluent (C).

Point 3: heart on the diaphragm

If we do not discipline ourselves to always use the inferior PVs as our reference point—and separate to the axial errors already described in lateral swings—we can miss an extremely serious anomaly concerning PVR. TAPVR is seen as either:

- associated with a complex cardiopathy like VAH (described earlier),[5] especially in those cases of right isomerism (Fig. 5.20; see also Fig. 5.8), or
- isolated but total,[12] posing a serious problem after birth, and even bringing on post- or neonatal death if there has been no diagnosis. Familial forms of this pathology exist, and here again we see the importance of the initial medical history which looks for a family history of surgery (most often in partial forms of the disease), or unexplained neonatal deaths (which could occur in undiagnosed complete forms of TAPVR) (Fig. 5.21). This research can be helped by Doppler, which is necessary in the case of a small LA but only after we are sure that the four-chamber view has been verified axially and is optimal.

Point 4: if we cannot distinguish the four chambers

In this situation we can identify the following:

Three chambers

Three chambers in the case of a UA or UV. The diagnosis of UA, frequently associated with AVSD, should not pose a particular problem in the total

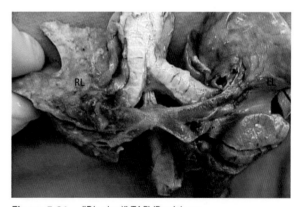

Figure 5.21 "Blocked" TAPVR with an above-diaphragmatic confluent finishing in the SVC. This newborn died at one month.

absence of an interauricular wall. This should lead us to search for Ellis–van Creveld syndrome (Fig. 5.22). There is *no* flap valve. The case of a UV is more delicate because of the difficulty in differentiating a UV from an extreme ventricular hypoplasia, in particular that of the left. In this case, the papillary muscle of the RV, which is large, is often mistaken as the IVS. But in these cases, careful analysis of the four-chamber view will not allow us to find balanced chambers with a normal crux of the heart.

Four+ chambers

Seeing a small, supplementary, rounded chamber at the left atrioventricular angle (Fig. 5.23; see also Fig 5.6) is witness to a most often dilated coronary sinus (CS) by a persistent left subclavian vein (LSCV). The importance of this dilatation and its eventual repercussions[13] depend on the association of the LSCV with an abnormal PVR found flowing there. Erroneous diagnoses of AVSD have been made in the case of a dilated CS in the presence of an imperfect four-chamber view (Fig. 5.24).[14]

Five chambers

We should be aware of the existence of a very rare doubling of the left atrial chamber: the triatrial heart. This "antechamber" receives the PV and is in communication with the LA by a tight orifice, which brings about the same effect as that of mitral stenosis with eventual repercussions on the development of the left tracts.

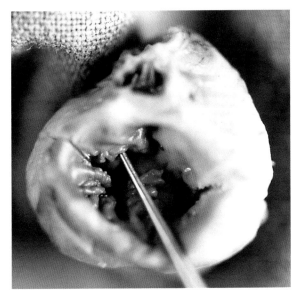

Figure 5.22   Right posterior view of the fetal heart with Ellis–van Creveld syndrome showing a UA overhanging a complete AVSD. Note the dysplasia of the bridging leaflets.

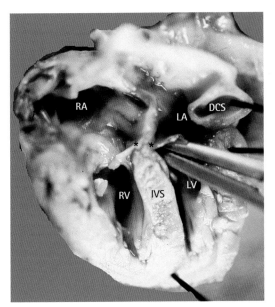

Figure 5.23   Macroscopic view of the four chambers with a dilated CS in trisomy 21. Note the LIAVV without defect (marked by *).

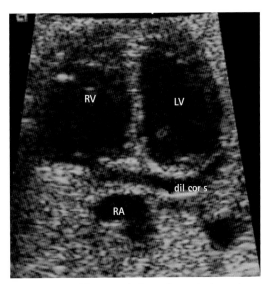

Figure 5.24   Ultrasound view of a posterior swing cutting a dilated CS. This can be mistaken for AVSD.

Point 5: asymmetric or discordant chambers

If the chambers are asymmetric we can distinguish a variety of architectural malformations

Right ventricular hypoplasia due to PA with IS (see Fig. 5.18) is found more often than tricuspid atresia (Fig. 5.25). In tricuspid atresia—certain cases have been published showing this condition to be associated with 22q11 deletion[15]—the right AV valve is closed but, due to the persistence of the bulbar ventricular foramen ensuring communication between the left and right outlet, the great vessels can be balanced. They are, however, often transposed.

With different degrees of severity and variable causes, left ventricular hypoplasia has a poor prognosis.[16] According to the level where the obstacle is found, the left chamber lumen will be seen (or not seen) and the left chamber wall might be hyperechogenic. Atresia or a tightening stenosis of the aorta creates an obstacle, the struggle against which causes fibroelastosis. This fibroelastosis can be seen as an hyperechogenicity.

Ebstein's anomalies (Fig. 5.27; see also Fig. 5.14) are associated with an often enlarged RA due to "atrialization" of the septal leaflet of the tricuspid valve. RV function can be very much reduced.

> ### !!! ATTENTION !!!
>
> A discreet asymmetry at a gestational age of 22 weeks has been described as a warning sign of coarctation of the aorta.[18] This pathology can be critical at birth. If there is the slightest suspicion, you should not hesitate to consult a pediatric cardiologist who can then follow the patient.

In cases where the chambers are discordant

An atrioventricular discordance is rare and defined as the communication between the RA and a ventricle of the left type (which has a smooth septum), while the left atrium (that which receives the PV) communicates with a ventricle of the right type (which has trabeculations). This anomaly, which is

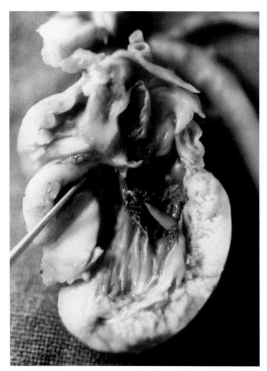

Figure 5.25 Tricuspid atresia seen within a macroscopic four-chamber view showing a dead-ended orifice.

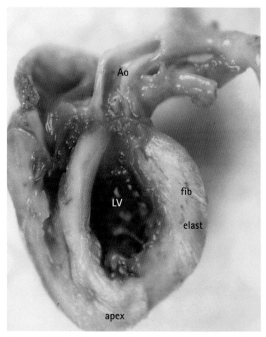

Figure 5.26 Macroscopic four-chamber view of the heart with aortic atresia and fibroelastosis.

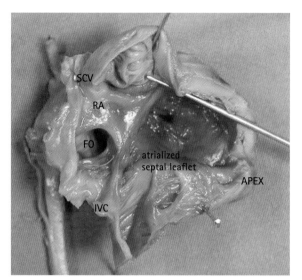

Figure 5.27   Macroscopic view of the heart with Ebstein's disease showing the right inlet tract open.

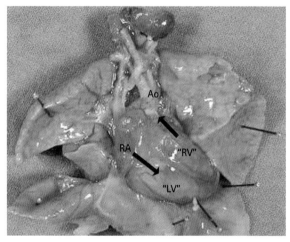

Figure 5.28   Macroscopic view of the HLB having a double discordance or "corrected transposition".

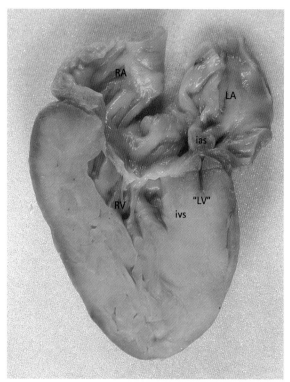

Figure 5.29   Macroscopic four-chamber view of a heart with mitral atresia.

Point 6: rings that are impermeable or not offset

The atrioventricular valves should be permeable. It is necessary to collect images of the four-chamber view with the valves closed and opened. They are impermeable in two pathologies: mitral (Fig. 5.29) or tricuspid (see Fig. 5.25) atresias.

The verification of the offsetting of the atrioventricular valves is an important step which should be part of the examination using the four-chamber view. In fact, the absence of offsetting, or the linear insertion of atrioventricular valves (LIAVV), is a marker common to all levels of the spectrum of AVSD. This spectrum goes from the continued persistence of the initial atrioventricular canal in the form of a complete AVSD (Figs 5.30 and 5.31) to the LIAVV without defect, which we have described both anatomically and through US.[20,21] This spectrum then passes through partial AVSD

relatively easy to appreciate in fetal pathology, is visible through a rigorous study of the atrioventricular concordance in the four-chamber view. A discordance that is visible in the inlet, and thus atrioventricular, will lead us to look for an associated ventriculoarterial discordance. This double discordance was called the "corrected TGV" (Fig. 5.28).[19] Theoretically, without any early or notable consequence, it is frequently associated with other pathologies—VSD, pulmonary stenosis, rhythm trouble—which justify the search for these concordances.

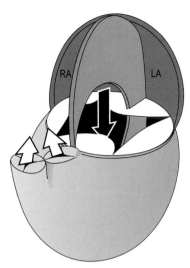

Figure 5.30   Embryological diagram of the "verticalized" heart seen from the left. The AVSD is still complete.

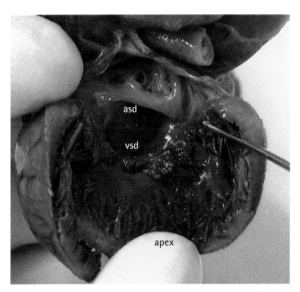

Figure 5.31   Macroscopic view of the "verticalized" heart. Opening of the left inlet showing a large defect with two bridging leaflets over the crest.

with the interatrial defect of the ostium primum type and mitral cleft, or a partial AVSD with an inlet defect. The close relationship between AVSD and trisomy 21 is well known (Fig. 5.32).

In the case of complete AVSD, the common valves, inferior and superior (Figs 5.33 and 5.34), bridge the AVSD from above. Dependent on the degree of severity within the spectrum, we can eventually visualize a septum intermedium which appears echogenic (Fig. 5.35). Sometimes the bridging leaflets are attached to the crest of the AVSD (Fig. 5.36). This takes into account the differences between the US aspect of the common valve without attachments (see Figs 5.33–5.35), opening and closing like a single wing of a seagull, and the attached bridging leaflet (Fig. 5.37; see also Fig. 5.36) which beats like the two wings of a seagull. (Fig. 5.38).

In the case of partial AVSD, a defect is described as either ASD of the ostium primum type, (Figs 5.39 and 5.40) or VSD of the inlet type (Figs 5.41 and 5.42). In both cases the atrioventricular leaflets appear to be inserted at the same level. There can be a mitral cleft, but here as well, there is *no* offsetting.

Next to partial AVSD with defects, we have described a minor form of AVSD, which we named the LIAVV without defect (Figs 5.43–5.45; see

also Fig. 5.23),[20] which can now be observed by US (Fig. 5.46).[21]

There is a lack of the normal offsetting. (Figs 5.47 and 5.48).

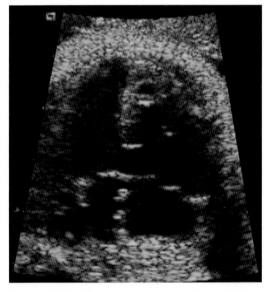

Figure 5.32   Ultrasound view of a trisomic 21 fetus. There is a complete AVSD in this apical incidence. Note the linear aspect of the bridging leaflet.

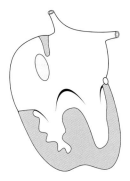

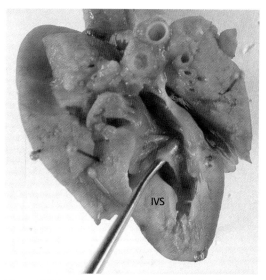

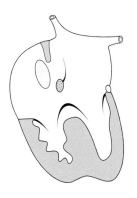

Figure 5.33 Diagram of a major form of complete AVSD.

Figure 5.34 Macroscopic view of a major form of complete AVSD with the probe under the bridging leaflet (the "one wing" of a seagull).

Figure 5.35 Diagram of a view of a complete AVSD with the septum intermedium.

In normal hearts, the offsetting of the atrioventricular valves is *constant*, whereas in *all* forms of the AVSD spectrum we observe a linear insertion of these atrioventricular valves which makes them look like the wings of a seagull (see Fig. 5.38).

A yet unpublished large prospective study has also shown that in certain CTCs we can find a LIAVV with defect. This confirms fetal pathologic observations that have been seen in these hearts (Fig. 5.49).

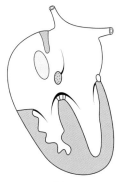

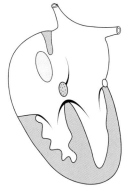

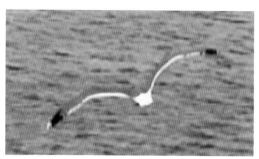

Figure 5.38 A seagull flying over the Mediterranean.

Figure 5.36 Diagram of a view of a complete AVSD with the septum intermedium and attached to the bridging leaflet on the crest of the VSD like two wings of a seagull.

Figure 5.37 Diagram of a view of a partial AVSD with an ASD ostium primum.

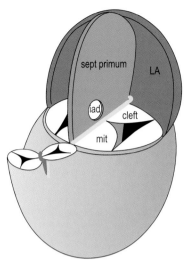

Figure 5.39 Embryological diagram seen from the left of a partial AVSD with ASD ostium primum. iad, interatrial defect.

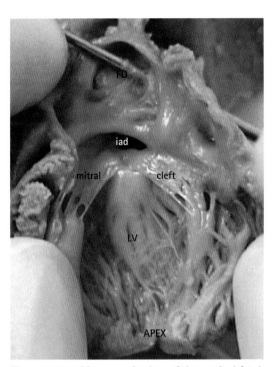

Figure 5.40 Macroscopic view of the vertical fetal heart opened to the left showing the ASD and mitral cleft. The probe passes through the "chicane" of the foramen ovale.

!!! ATTENTION !!!

Before concluding that there is an inlet anomaly, an asymmetry or an abnormal insertion of the valves, you must be certain—and clearly confirm—that the four-chamber view is strictly axial and situated at the optimal level.

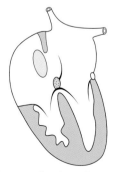

Figure 5.41 Diagram of a view of a partial AVSD with an inlet VSD.

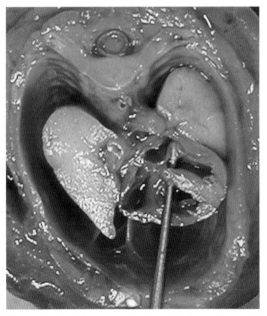

Figure 5.42 Macroscopic view of a HLB with an inlet VSD (probe) of a partial AVSD in a trisomic 21 fetus.

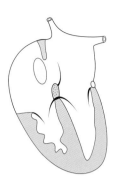

Figure 5.43   Diagram of LIAVV without defect.

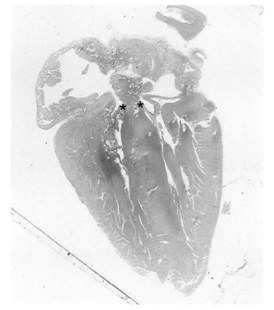

Figure 5.45   Histologic view of the four chambers of a fetal heart with trisomy 21 and LIAVV without defect. The septal leaflets insert (*) at the same level.

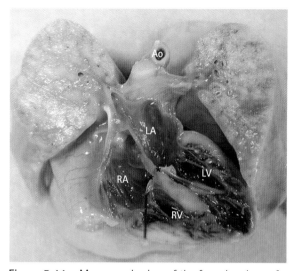

Figure 5.44   Macroscopic view of the four chambers of a fetal heart with trisomy 21 and LIAVV without defect. Note the ballooning septal tricuspid leaflet (marked by *).

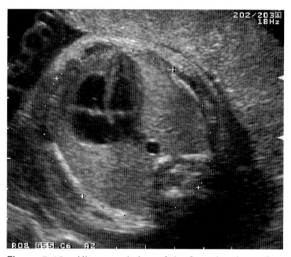

Figure 5.46   Ultrasound view of the four chambers of a fetal heart with trisomy 21 and LIAVV without defect. Note the ballooning septal tricuspid leaflet.

There are two criteria for assuring the quality of this view which should be visualized on the same image plane. They are:

- The arrival of the two inferior PVs in the LA.
- The visualization of one (or two) complete rib(s) depending on the incidence.

At the level of the TAD and the optimal four-chamber view, the presence of at least one complete rib confirms the axial nature of the view.

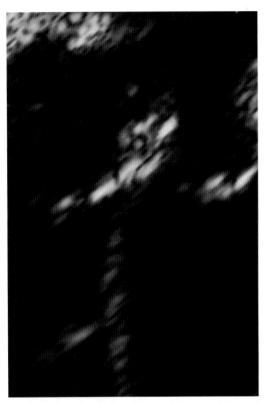

Figure 5.47 Crux of the heart with normal offsetting in an US scan.

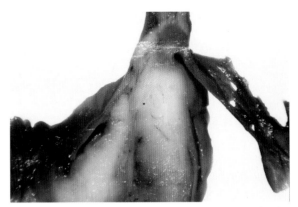

Figure 5.48 Crux of the heart with normal offsetting in macroscopy.

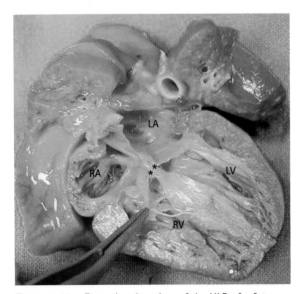

Figure 5.49 Four-chamber view of the HLB of a fetus with tetralogy of Fallot. Note there is a LIAVV (marked by *). The defect is seen in the outlet.

THIRD STEP. PATHOLOGIES OF THE OUTLET

Often outlet pathologies are suspected due to certain small warning signs observed on the four-chamber view. These include:

- A right descending aorta (see Figs 5.6–5.8).
- The axis of the heart at 60° (see Figs 5.6 and 5.15), with balanced ventricular outlet chambers, and a heart in the form of a "boot" as seen in severe forms of tetralogy of Fallot.

At the outlet level these different pathologies touch each of the key points, which include:

- **Point 7:** two balanced outlet chambers separated by an outlet septum with an intact, normal alignment.
- **Point 8:** two crossed vessels.
- **Point 9:** outlet tracts that are balanced and concordant.
- **Point 10:** a regular aortic arch.

Point 7: pathology

The presence of a defect of the alignment in the outlet septum is a direct warning sign of CTC. If the defect is situated on the trabeculated outlet section of the IVS (Fig. 5.50) it is essentially a VSD with a misalignment, which destroys the septal–aortic continuity at the level of the junction between the muscle of the IVS and the fibrous aortic wall.

This type of large outlet VSD (Figs 5.51 and 5.52) is characteristic of CTCs and is the most

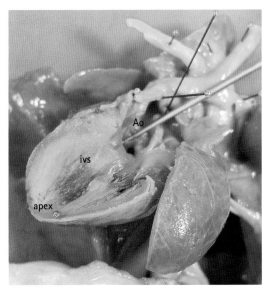

Figure 5.50   The fetal heart opened to the left. The probe pushes along the aortic wall into the right ventricle.

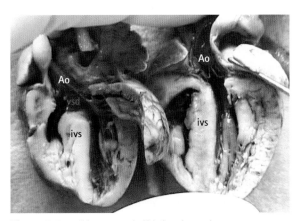

Figure 5.51   Macroscopic LV–Ao views: large misalignment VSD in a tetralogy of Fallot with an overriding aorta compared to a normal heart.

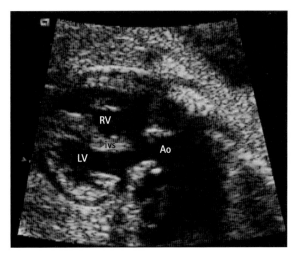

Figure 5.52   Ultrasound view of a large overriding aorta.

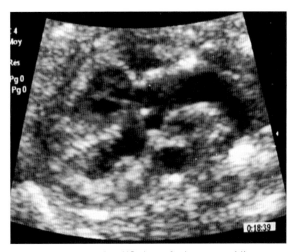

Figure 5.53   Another US view of a large overriding aorta.

frequent type of VSD associated with CTC. If it is associated with an anterior swing of the conal septum, depending on the degree of swing, it can result in different forms of tetralogy of Fallot through to PA with OS (Fig. 5.53).

Far rarer is a VSD of CTC involving the infundibular septum, which is smaller and more difficult to see, except in the "SOS" view, which is what we call the sagittal LV–Ao view. Infundibular VSDs are situated at a distance from the membranous septum and are more often associated with CTC caused by a posterior swing. (Fig. 5.54) The milder forms are coarctation syndromes (narrowing of the aorta associated with an outlet VSD); major forms are interruption of the aorta. When the VSD is not seen right away, an asymmetry of the great vessels when the admission chambers are balanced should draw us to this region, allowing us to discern this defect.

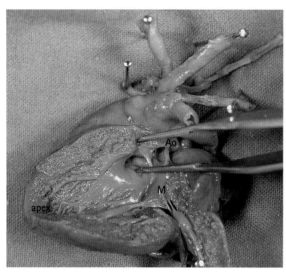

Figure 5.54   Lateral left view of the outlet tract. An infundibulum VSD is more frequent in cases of a posterior swing. Note the crest situated between the forceps which forms an obstacle to the aortic outlet.

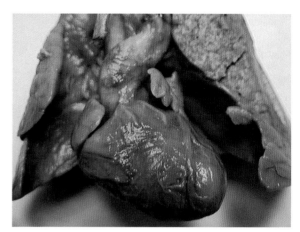

Figure 5.55   Fetal HLB with CAT. Note the "boot" shape of the heart responsible for the 60° axis.

Constant VSD in conotruncal cardiopathies is for the most part caused by misalignment.

> Verifying septal–aortic continuity and the balance of vessels (having the same diameter) eliminates the possibility of a large majority of the CTC spectrum, especially the most common or severe types, such as tetralogy of Fallot, and PA with OS.

As in AVSD, there is a CTC malformation spectrum. Faced with each and every form of CTC we should research the possibility of a 22q11 deletion if the standard karyotype is normal.[22]

The major form of this spectrum is the persistence of the common arterial trunk (CAT) (Fig. 5.55) where the infundibular or conal septum is absent; a unique outlet vessel overrides the VSD. The PT arises from the CAT soon after the ring, which is frequently displastic.

Other CTCs are differentiated by size and position of the great vessels relative to the VSD:

- The minor form is an isolated outlet VSD.
- In the case of an anterior swing (Fig. 5.56) of the conal or infundibular septum, and depending

on the degree of this swing, we move from a minor to a major form of tetralogy of Fallot. At the extreme end is PA with OS. These cardiopathies are very frequent in fetal pathology, where they are seen to evolve,[23] and represent 55% of cases of CTC.

- In the case of a posterior swing (Fig. 5.57), the aortic flow is seen to proportionally diminish at the degree of the swing with stenosis (in minor forms) to interruptions (major forms) of certain sections of the aortic arch. This can be explained by the multiple and specific embryonic origins of these different segments. The minor form is the coarctation syndrome which associates a partial stenosis (or coarctation of the aorta) with an outlet VSD. The major form occurs when the aortic arch is interrupted (IAA) (Fig. 5.58), which itself exists in several forms (about 14% of fetal CTC, but it is associated in 80% of cases of 22q11 deletion where the IAA has been visualized as being of the B type).[22] This form of IAA is characterized by the interruption (illustrated by the dotted lines in Figure 5.58) occurring between the left primitive carotid artery and the left subclavian artery. (Fig. 5.59) In IAA attention should be given to the "vertical" aspect of the ascending aorta before the interruption of its arch.
- In anomalies involving asymmetry in the size of the vessels we can add the variable degree involved

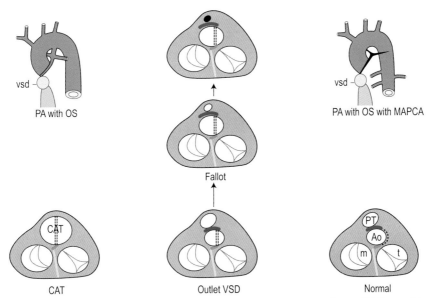

Figure 5.56   Diagram of the CTC spectrum caused by an anterior swing: From tetralogy of Fallot to PA with OS.

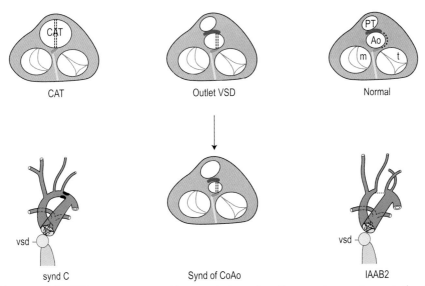

Figure 5.57   Diagram of the CTC spectrum caused by a posterior swing: From syndrome of coarctation to interruption of the aortic arch (IAA).

in malpositioning of these vessels above the IVS. These positional errors can be of such importance that it is difficult to differentiate a tetralogy of Fallot in which less than 50% of the aorta receives a flow from the RV from a double outlet right ventricle in which the PT and the aorta primarily exit out of the RV.

Certain particularities of CTC chiefly evoke a 22q11 deletion: a right aortic arch; a type B2 IAA (see Fig. 5.58); the presence of main aorto-pulmonary collateral arteries (MAPCA) (Fig. 5.60) in PA with OS; and an absence of the ductus arteriosus (DA). In addition, 30% of fetuses present with associated renal anomalies.[22]

!!! ATTENTION !!!

The discovery of an outlet cardiopathy in a fetus with a standard normal karyotype in the context of oligohydramnios leads us immediately to consider 22q11 deletion because 30% are associated with a renal anomaly.

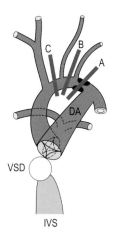

Figure 5.59 Diagram of the different levels of IAA.

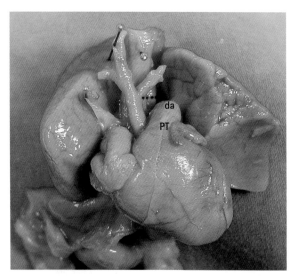

Figure 5.58 Heart–lung block showing a type B IAA. Note the steepness of the ascending aorta and the absence of continuity between the primitive left carotid and the arterial canal.

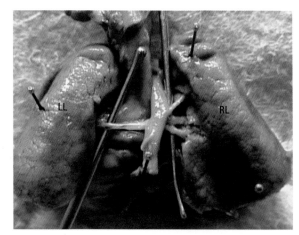

Figure 5.60 Posterior view of a HLB in a PA with OS. MAPCA coming out of the aorta to the right and the left lungs.

Point 8: the verification of the crossing over of the great vessels is a critical moment

It is here that we can allay suspicion of a complete TGV—an obsession of the fetal US practitioner. TGV occurs in an otherwise normal fetus whose prognosis depends on the prenatal diagnosis of this cardiopathy.[24,25] Anatomically, TGV is described as ventriculoarterial discordance (Figs 5.61 and 5.62). The origin of the aorta occurs in the RV, more anterior than the PT in the LV at the center of the heart. This results in an almost parallel direction of the two vessels (Fig. 5.63) as they proceed towards their junction with the descending aorta (Figs 5.64 and 5.65).

The US diagnosis of TGV means that we must check the emergence of the vessels from each ventricle, noting that:

- Out of the LV comes a vessel which will rejoin the descending aorta and rapidly divide, thus it is the PT.
- Out of the anterior RV emerges a vessel which joins the descending aorta after a long antero-posterior trajectory (Fig. 5.66). This vessel gives rise to the vessels of the neck, thus it is an aorta.

An isolated right or left ventriculo-arterial discordance is a vital clue to orient our diagnosis towards that of TGV.

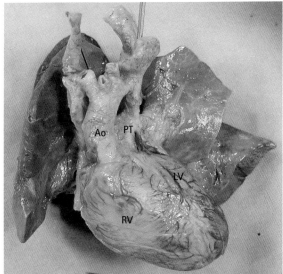

Figure 5.61   Macroscopic view of TGV.

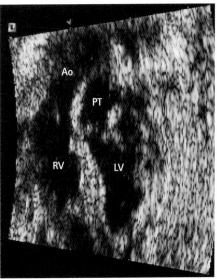

Figure 5.62   Ultrasound incidence in TGV.

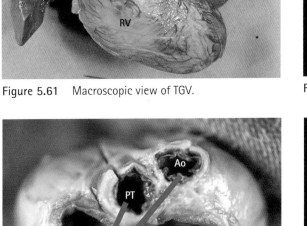

Figure 5.63   Right posterior view of a heart after ablation of the auricles and the great vessels. Arrows indicate the trajectory of the vessels in rejoining the descending aorta in TGV.

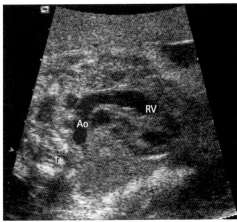

Figure 5.64   Ultrasound incidence in TGV. A view close to the three-vessel view (3VT).

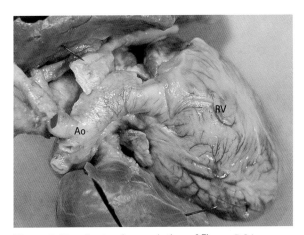

Figure 5.65   Anatomic correlation of Figure 5.64.

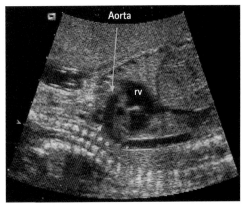

Figure 5.66   Ultrasound incidence in TGV. Sagittal, the aorta is seen to begin not in the center of the heart but in a ventricle situated behind the sternum.

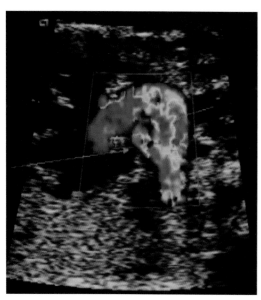

Figure 5.67 Large aorta, small PA. Tetralogy of Fallot. Look for the outlet VSD.

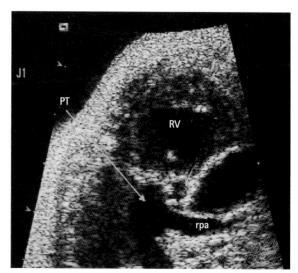

Figure 5.68 Ductus arteriosus view. Large PT, small aorta. If the four-chamber view is in equilibrium look for a VSD (CTC by posterior swing). If the four-chamber view is not in equilibrium verify if there is a hypoplasia of the left tracts.

Point 9: a lack of balance can involve several elements

A lack of balance between the chambers

This might already have been seen on the four-chamber view when we paid attention to checking the permeability of the atrioventricular rings. This is the case in left tract hypoplasias (see Figs 5.12 and 5.13) which are more frequent than those concerning the right hypoplasias (Figs 5.16 and 5.17).

Vessel imbalance

Though seen while viewing a single vessel—e.g. a large arch, a small PT (Fig. 5.67), or one that is not seen at all—it is often better appreciated when observing two vessels on the same image, the arterial duct view (Fig. 5.68) or the three-vessel view. This imbalance makes searching for an outlet VSD a priority, which, if found, leads us to a diagnosis of CTC.

In studying vessel imbalance through the three-vessel view it is important to appreciate the direction of flow of the two vessels in Doppler; this is essential in certain cardiopathies called duct-dependent. Normally both the aortic and DA flow is directed towards the descending aorta. This vascularization, which ends with the physiologic

closing of the DA in the hours following birth, is called duct-dependent. This problem is one for the pediatric cardiologists but its US visualization is relatively simple.

The confirmation of convergent flow of aorta and DA in the three-vessel view is essential. A reverse flow is always pathologic, indicating a retrograde vascularization of the PT or the Ao.

Point 10: irregular aortic arch

We have already spoken of large arches which are noticeable in different forms of tetralogy of Fallot where they are associated with VSD. Though the irregularities of the aortic arch are subtle, they can eventually be examined using the three-vessel view.

Coarctations of the isthmus of the aorta is a pathology that often becomes critical with the closing of the arterial duct. This pathology is difficult to recognize by direct signs but can be suspected due to its effects on the hemodynamics. This causes a type of ventricular asymmetry, noted at a gestational age of 22 weeks in the absence of any other pathology.[18]

Coarctation of the horizontal aorta is characteristic of Turner's syndrome (karyotype primarily 45X0).

Attention

Do not confuse coarctations with the syndromes of coarctation CTC caused by a posterior swing of the conal septum, which are always associated with a VSD.

The third step necessitates static and dynamic studies based on multiple views that are complementary, which include the measurement of the diameters of the great vessels.

References

1. Acharya G, Sitras V, Maltau JM et al. Major congenital heart disease in Northern Norway: shortcomings of pre- and postnatal diagnosis. Acta Obstet Gynecol Scand 2004; 83(12):1124–1129.
2. Maclean K, Dunwoodie SL. Breaking symmetry: a clinical overview of left–right patterning. Clin Genet 2004; 65(6):6441–6457.
3. Pasquini L, Tan T, Yen Ho S, Gardiner H. The implications for fetal outcome of an abnormal arrangement of the abdominal vessels. Cardiol Young 2005; 15(1):135–142.
4. Machado-Atias I, Anselmi G, Machado-Hernandez I, Febres C. Discordances between the different types of atrial arrangement and the positions of the thoraco-abdominal organs. Cardiol Young 2001; 11(5):5543–5550.
5. Wessels MW, Frohn-Mulder IM, Cromme-Dijkhuis AH, Wladimiroff JW. In utero diagnosis of infra-diaphragmatic total anomalous pulmonary venous return. Ultrasound Obstet Gynecol 1996; 8(3):206–209.
6. Lin JH, Chang CI, Wang JK et al. Intrauterine diagnosis of heterotaxy syndrome. Am Heart J 2002; 143(6):1002–1008.
7. Huggon IC, Cook AC, Smeeton NC et al. Atrioventricular septal defects diagnosed in fetal life: associated cardiac and extra-cardiac abnormalities and outcome. J Am Coll Cardiol 2000; 36(2):593–601.
8. Yoo SJ, Lee YH, Kim ES et al. Tetralogy of Fallot in the fetus: findings at targeted sonography. Ultrasound Obstet Gynecol 1999; 14(1):29–37.
9. Shipp TD, Bromley B, Hornberger LK et al. Levorotation of the fetal cardiac axis: a clue for the presence of congenital heart disease. Obstet Gynecol 1995; 85(1):97–102.
10. Daubeney PE, Delany DJ, Anderson RH et al. for the United Kingdom and Ireland Collaborative Study of Pulmonary Atresia with Intact Ventricular Septum. Pulmonary atresia with intact ventricular septum: range of morphology in a population-based study. J Am Coll Cardiol 2002; 39(10):1670–1679.
11. Khoshhal S, Sandor GG, Duncan WJ. Pulmonary atresia with intact ventricular septum and antenatal left ventricular failure. Cardiol Young 2004; 14(3):335–337.
12. Allan LD, Sharland GK. The echocardiographic diagnosis of totally anomalous pulmonary venous connection in the fetus. Heart 2001; 85(4):433–437.
13. Jouannic JM, Picone O, Martinovic J et al. Diminutive fetal left ventricle at mid-gestation associated with persistent left superior vena cava and coronary sinus dilatation. Ultrasound Obstet Gynecol 2003; 22(5):527–530.
14. Chaoui R, Heling KS, Kalache KD. Caliber of the coronary sinus in fetuses with cardiac defects with and without left persistent superior vena cava and in growth-restricted fetuses with heart-sparing effect. Prenat Diagn 2003; 23(7):552–557.
15. Marino B, Digilio MC, Novelli G et al. Tricuspid atresia and 22q11 deletion. Am J Med Genet 1997; .
16. Mahle WT, Clancy RR, McGaurn SP et al. Impact of prenatal diagnosis on survival and early neurologic morbidity in neonates with the hypoplastic left heart syndrome. Pediatrics 2001; 107(6):1277–1282.
17. Sharland GK, Chita SK, Fagg NL et al. Left ventricular dysfunction in the fetus: relation to aortic valve anomalies and endocardial fibroelastosis. Br Heart J 1991; 66(6):419–424.
18. David N, Iselin M, Blaysat G et al. Disproportion in diameter of the cardiac chambers and great arteries in the fetus. Contribution to the prenatal diagnosis of coarctation of the aorta. Arch Mal Coeur Vaiss 1997; 90(5):673–678. In French.
19. Sharland G, Tingay R, Jones A, Simpson JM. Atrioventricular and ventriculoarterial discordance (congenitally corrected transposition of the great arteries): echocardiographic features, associations, and outcome in 34 fetuses. Heart 2005; 91(11):1453–1458; epub Mar 10, 2005.
20. Fredouille C, Piercecchi-Marti MD, Liprandi A et al. Linear insertion of atrioventricular valves without septal defect: a new anatomical landmark for Down's syndrome? Fetal Diagn Ther 2002; 17(3):188–192. Erratum in: Fetal Diagn Ther 2002; 17(5):292.
21. Fredouille C, Baschet N, Morice JE et al. Linear insertion of the atrioventricular valves without defect. Arch Mal Coeur Vaiss 2005; 98(5):549–555. In French.
22. Boudjemline Y, Fermont L, Le Bidois J et al. Prevalence of 22q11 deletion in fetuses with conotruncal cardiac defects: a 6-year prospective study. J Pediatr 2001; 138(4):520–524.
23. Pepas LP, Savis A, Jones A et al. An echographic study of tetralogy of Fallot in the fetus and infant. Cardiol Young 2003; 13(3):240–247.
24. Yates RS. The influence of prenatal diagnosis on postnatal outcome in patients with structural congenital heart disease. Prenat Diagn 2004; 24(13):1143–1149.
25. Jouannic JM, Gavard L, Fermont L et al. Sensitivity and specificity of prenatal features of physiological shunts to predict neonatal clinical status in transposition of the great arteries. Circulation 2004; 110(13):1743–1746; epub Sep 13, 2004.

Chapter **6**

When: fetal morphological examination after the discovery of a cardiopathy

by Catherine Fredouille

When a cardiac anomaly has been discovered, the ultrasound (US) specialist must concentrate on finding associated morphological anomalies in order to better orient the diagnosis. This research can be guided by the type of cardiopathy.

In the absence of a known karyotype, we first look for markers associated with chromosomal anomalies. The practice of finding an early abnormal karyotype for an excess of nuchal translucency (NT) or an alarming serum marker has changed our possibilities in this area.

It is now usual to practice morphological US in the context of a known normal karyotype,[1] which is why we extend our research to US markers of certain genetic syndromes and associations. With this in mind, besides concentrating on those organs normally examined through morphological US, we can extend our research towards specific signs, which are rarer but whose discovery will modify the prognosis.

!!! ATTENTION !!!

Attention should be paid to the limitations of an US examination: it may display certain dysmorphic elements *poorly* and will *never* reveal the possibility of mental retardation.

TWO POSSIBILITIES EXIST

THE KARYOTYPE IS UNKNOWN

We first consider a situation that occurs for the patient who did not have—or refused—an early US investigation and/or the investigation of serum markers (as in a twin pregnancy). This is also true in the case where the initial results happened to be normal. In all such cases, the discovery of a cardiac anomaly during US at a gestational age of 22 weeks—or even 32 weeks—requires us first to look for those signs associated with the principal chromosomal abnormalities.

> Even when this morphological study is negative, when we are faced with the discovery of a cardiopathy, we must *systematically* propose the determination of the karyotype. This should be associated with an investigation of 22q11 chromosomal deletion if it is a conotruncal cardiopathy (CTC).

Warning signs of chromosomal anomalies[1,2]

In order of frequency, these are as follows.

Trisomy 21 (T21; Down's syndrome)

This occurs in 1 in 700 pregnancies (Fig. 6.1).

Despite the increase in the early diagnosis of this pathology, certain women—voluntarily or otherwise—have not had early tests for this condition. In questioning the patient, we should seek out elements to help direct our research: an old or very young maternal age; an inadequate dating for the US; serum markers not performed; or a NT not taken into account or practiced before 11 gestational weeks, after 14 gestational weeks, or a NT that was seen to be normal.

The type of cardiopathy can point us in the right direction. It is often primarily a cardiopathy of the atrioventricular septal defect (AVSD) spectrum, whether complete AVSD (Figs 6.2 and 6.3) to linear insertion of atrioventricular valves (LIAVV) without defect (Figs 6.4 and 6.5);[3,4] trisomy 21 should also be considered with tetralogy of Fallot.

The examination looks for extracardiac anomalies or malformations:[5,6] a flat profile with shortening

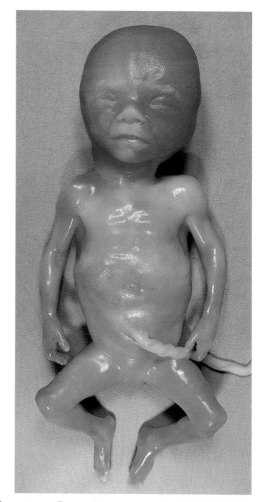

Figure 6.1   Fetus with trisomy 21.

or even the absence of the fetal nasal bone (FNB) and a filling of the small nasofrontal space; small ears; a thick nape of the neck or nuchal thickening (Fig. 6.6); a brachy- and even an amesophalangy of the fifth digit (Fig. 6.7); and a spacing of the big toe (Fig. 6.8). All these characteristics are more evocative than images of a pyelectasis, a suspicion of esophageal atresia (Fig. 6.9), or a unique umbilical artery (UUA).

Trisomy 18 (T18; Edwards' syndrome)

This occurs in 1 in 1800 pregnancies.

Trisomy 18 is more often associated with outlet cardiopathies; it is first considered when the cardiopathy (Fig. 6.10)[6] is associated with intrauterine retarded growth (IURG) (Fig. 6.11). Nearly

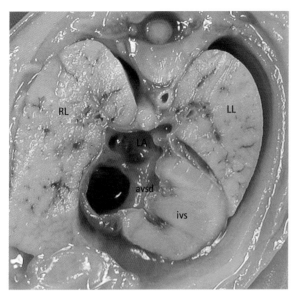

Figure 6.2 Anatomic thoracic four-chamber view: complete AVSD. The interventricular septum (IVS) is short and thick.

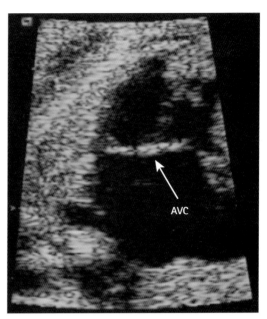

Figure 6.3 An apical incidence of a complete AVSD. The common leaflet is linear.

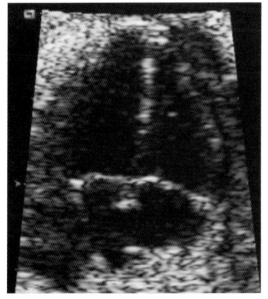

Figure 6.4 Apical four-chamber view of a LIAVV without defect. There is no offsetting.

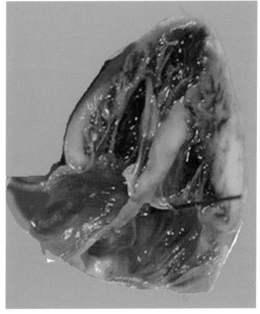

Figure 6.5 Apical anatomic four-chamber view of a LIAVV without defect. The needle is under the septal tricuspid leaflet which is not stuck to the IVS.

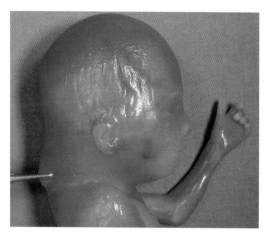

Figure 6.6 Trisomy 21 (T21) showing the thick neck (nuchal thickening).

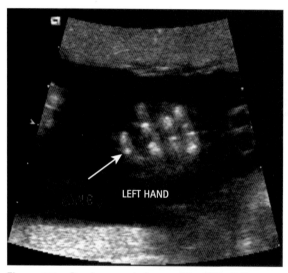

LEFT HAND

Figure 6.7 Brachymesophalangy of the fifth digit.

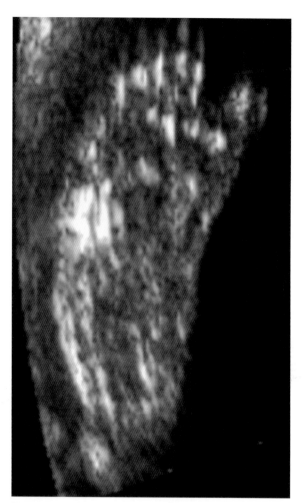

Figure 6.8 Spread of the large toe.

always present, IURG should not always be attributed to a possible coexistent vascular pathology.

The discovery of clenched hands (Figs 6.12 and 6.13) (with the impossibility of obtaining an image with the hands open), an aplasia of the radial ray responsible for "boot hands", a small exomphalos, spina bifida, or a diaphragmatic hernia all lead us to this diagnosis. But as in all chromosomal anomalies there exist minor forms of this pathology which support the principle of systematically asking for a karyotype faced with *any and all* cardiopathies.

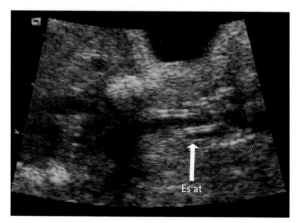

Es at

Figure 6.9 Proximal part of esophagus in esophageal atresia.

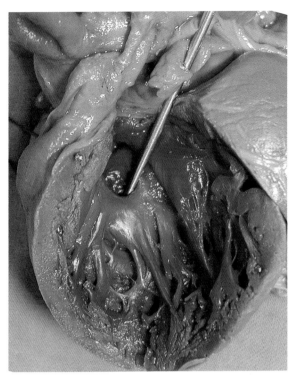

Figure 6.10   Open heart positioned vertically. The probe is in an outlet VSD in a T18 fetus.

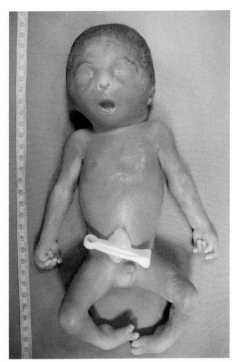

Figure 6.11   Week 27 of a T18 pregnancy. The fetus has the development of only 24 weeks demonstrating IURG. Notice the dysmorphia, the clenched hands, and the club-foot.

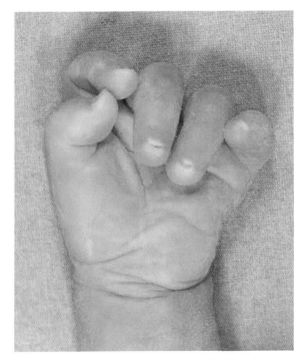

Figure 6.12   Macroscopic view of clenched hands.

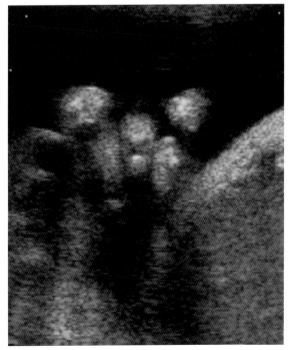

Figure 6.13   Ultrasound view of clenched hands.

Trisomy 13 (T13; Patau's syndrome)

This occurs in 1 in 5000 pregnancies.

The pathognomonic triad of a labiopalatine cleft (Fig. 6.14), holoprosencephaly (Fig. 6.15), and hexadactyly (Figs 6.16 and 6.17) is not always seen together. In the absence of all of these signs the diagnosis can be directed by the type of cardiopathy: frequency of the AVSD or a common arterial trunk (CAT) with displastic valves (hyperechogenic).

Next to these three frequent anomalies—whose minor forms we should be aware of—two other anomalies seldom go unnoticed at 12 gestational

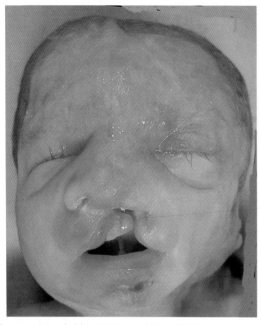

Figure 6.14   Labiopalatine cleft in a T13 fetus.

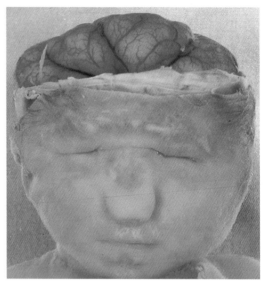

Figure 6.15   A lobar holoprosencephaly in a T13 fetus. Notice the microphthalmos, the unique naris, and the small mouth. This demonstrates the saying that the "face reflects the brain".

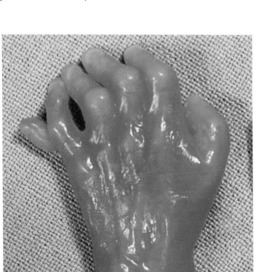

Figure 6.16   Macroscopic view of hexadactyly in a T13 fetus.

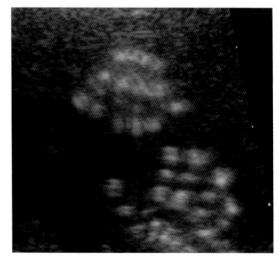

Figure 6.17   Ultrasound view of hexadactyly in a T13 fetus.

weeks. More than NT (Fig. 6.18), we often have to deal with a hygroma with anasarca in Turner's syndrome or a very early IUGR in triploidy.

Turner's syndrome

Turner's syndrome (Fig. 6.19) is with a karyotype primarily of 45X0. Its early diagnosis is frequently made when faced with a hygroma which can be differentiated from an augmentation of the NT at 12 gestational weeks. This could be a description of hydrops with anasarca. The diagnosis of the characteristic cardiopathy will only be made in fetal pathology; it is a stenosis of the horizontal section of the aorta in a female fetus (Fig. 6.20). Approximately 95% of pregnancies with a fetus having 45X0 are spontaneously interrupted and stillborn.

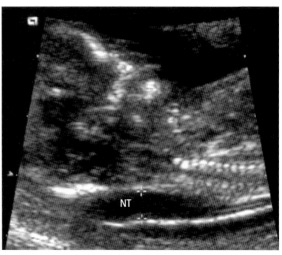

Figure 6.18   Nuchal translucency.

Triploidy

This is a pathology which is often proposed when we see an early, major form of IURG, and which is frequently taken to be an error of dating at the beginning of pregnancy. We note that there is often a disproportion between the head and the body, thin members with a large head (Fig. 6.21). In certain forms, we equally observe a highly suggestive fetus–placenta disequilibrium. Here, associated with a severe type of CTC in the form of a tetralogy of Fallot (Fig. 6.22), we see syndactyly III–IV (Fig. 6.23), characteristic, but difficult to see on US.

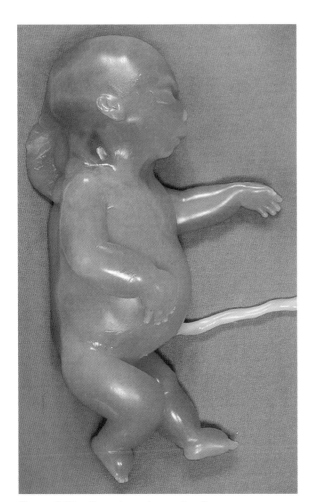

Figure 6.19   Turner's syndrome showing Bonnevie–Ullrich syndrome (hygroma, anasarca, and generalized edema) with primarily a 45X0 karyotype.

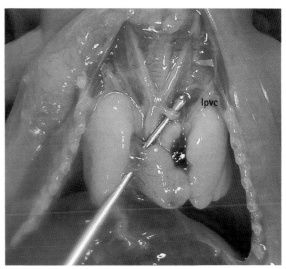

Figure 6.20   Fetal heart–lung block (HLB) showing horizontal aortic arch stenosis, which is typical of Turner's syndrome. Notice the left persistent caval vein.

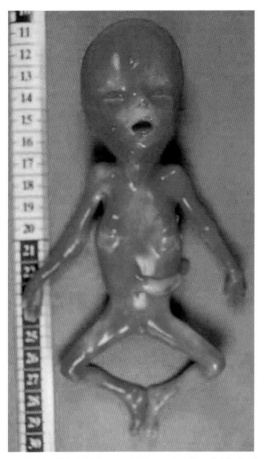

Figure 6.21   Triploid fetus with large head and thin limbs.

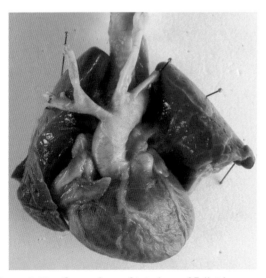

Figure 6.22   Severe form of tetralogy of Fallot in a triploid fetus.

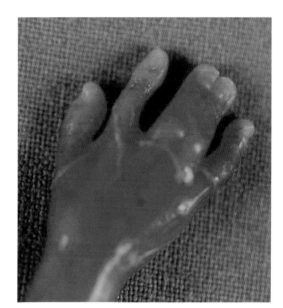

Figure 6.23   III–IV typical syndactyly.

THE KARYOTYPE IS KNOWN TO BE NORMAL

This situation is becoming more frequent.[7] Attention should be paid to two elements.

First, the karyotype can be made using a culture from different cells (biopsy of the trophoblast, cells from the amniotic liquid, or fetal blood) which can produce discordance in the results, for example by disregarding a tetrasomy 12p in a fetus appearing quite similar to Fryns' syndrome (Figs 6.24 and 6.25). (If the karyotype seems to be normal in fetal blood, the tetrasomy appears only when requested on an investigation of the amniotic fluid.)

In addition, certain minor pathologies of the karyotype can only be suspected after a re-examination of the initial karyotype, made after the discovery of a cardiopathy. Finally, an indication for specific research such as exploring a 4p deletion, for instance (Fig. 6.26), or even the possibility of a new karyotype, can be considered.

Second, the "standard" karyotype only explores the chromosomal pathologies of number. The discovery of a CTC leads us to request a complementary research in the 22q11 chromosomal deletion. This deletion will primarily be found in cases of IAA of the B type (Fig. 6.27), or with a pulmonary atresia with opened septum (PA with OS) with aortic–pulmonary collaterals (or main aorta–

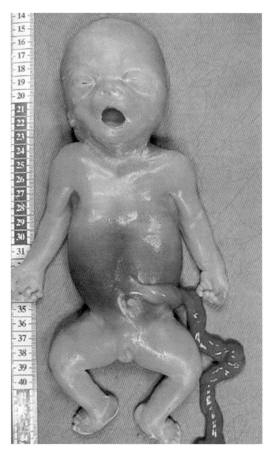

Figure 6.24   Fetus having a normal karyotype in fetal blood suspected of having Fryns' syndrome.

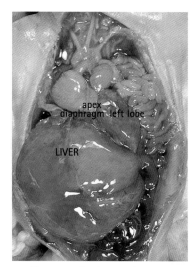

Figure 6.25   The same fetus as in Figure 6.24 with the viscera showing a diaphragmatic hernia. A new karyotype carried out using the amniotic fluid showed a 12p tetrasomy.

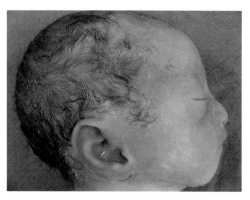

Figure 6.26   A fetus with 4p deletion having a profile "like a Greek helmet".

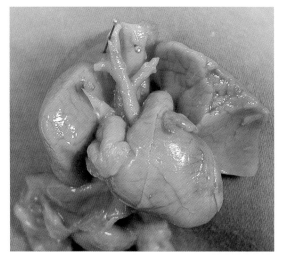

Figure 6.27   Anterior view of a HLB IAA type B in a 22q11 deletion.

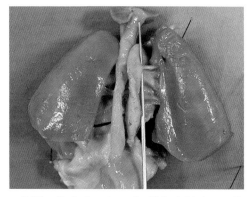

Figure 6.28   Posterior view of a HLB: right descending aorta with MAPCA under the probe in a 22q11 deletion.

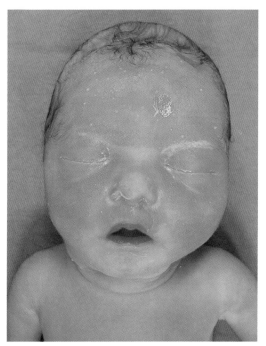

Figure 6.29   Light dysmorphia in a 22q11 deletion.

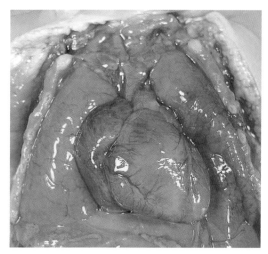

Figure 6.30   Thymus aplasia in a 22q11 deletion.

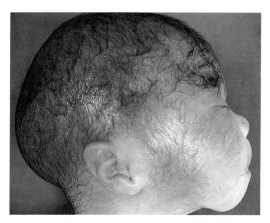

Figure 6.31   Profile of a fetus with fetal alcohol syndrome: long, smooth, and curved philtrum.

pulmonary collateral arteries: MAPCA), or even a CTC with a right aortic arch (Fig. 6.28) and/or the absence of the ductus arteriosus (DA). We equally find other anomalies: athymism; cleft palate or cleft lips; or frequent renal anomalies (in 29% of the cases),[8] which can rapidly hamper the examination by creating oligohydramnios. The dysmorphism (Fig. 6.29) is difficult to appreciate, except in those instances where there is a cleft. As for a thymic hypoplasia, it is easier to appreciate on the fetal–pathologic examination (Fig. 6.30) than with US.[9]

When we are sure of the absence of any chromosomal anomalies, then all associated markers, no matter how minor, should alert us to the possibility of a polymalformation syndrome, which radically modifies the prognosis.[10]

> Protocols when faced with a curable cardiopathy are very different depending on whether it is (or is not) part of a syndrome or association.

A cardiopathy associated with IURG, especially in the case where the NT is abnormal and the fetal karyotype is normal, leads to the following considerations.

Fetal alcohol syndrome[11]

Fetal alcohol syndrome must be considered when the practitioner is faced with a specific fetal profile: a long, smooth, and curved philtrum (Fig. 6.31). The mental prognosis is highly negative; the social and familial context can fool you.

Smith–Lemli–Opitz syndrome (SLOS)

This condition is an autosomal recessive (AR) syndrome. In searching for other signs that can be detectable by US,[12] other than IURG, sexual ambiguity should be examined in a fetus having a karyotype 46XY where the external sex is ambiguous, even feminine (Fig. 6.32). Look for anomalies of the extremities (Fig. 6.33), which are easier to see than dysmorphia (Fig. 6.34), where certain elements such as a short, wide neck are the consequence of an elevated NT.

The diagnosis of SLOS is possible by the analysis of cholesterol precursors in the amniotic fluid.[13] We should consider requesting it when faced with the association of a cardiopathy, IURG, hypogenitalism, and extremity anomalies. The interest in confirming this diagnosis is that SLOS is an AR syndrome, recurring once every four times, and we could practice this bioassay analysis at the beginning of the following pregnancy.

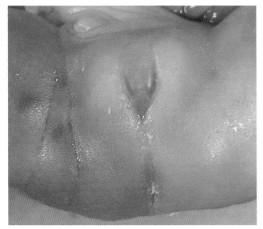

Figure 6.32   Hypogenitalism in a fetus with a 46XY karyotype.

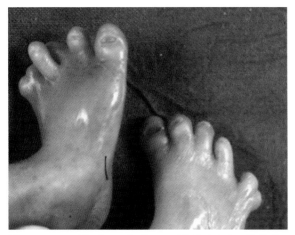

Figure 6.33   The feet of a fetus with Smith–Lemli–Opitz syndrome (SLOS).

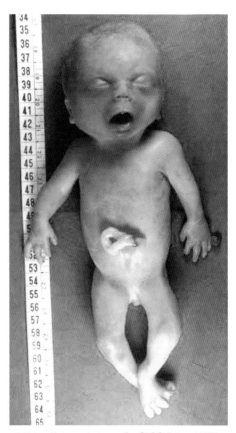

Figure 6.34   External view of a SLOS fetus 46XY: sex reversal, dysmorphia with a short, thick neck, and abnormalities of the limbs.

The CHARGE association[14]

CHARGE stands for:

Coloboma, which is not detectable by US
Heart (Fig. 6.35), for cardiac malformation
Atresia choanae, which can cause hydramnios (Fig. 6.36)
Retarded growth (often postnatal)
Genitals, e.g. hypospadias in a boy
Ears, anomalies of (Fig. 6.37); the external ears are asymmetric with the absence of the semicircular canals.

A diagnosis of CHARGE should be considered when we are faced with any curable cardiopathy, especially if associated with a sign such as a cleft lip and/or palate (Fig. 6.38), because of the severity of mental retardation, which is always prsent in this pathology.

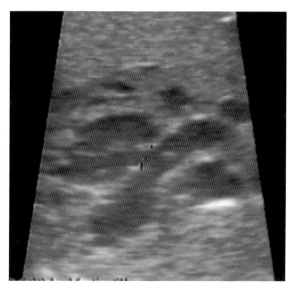

Figure 6.35 CHARGE association: small VSD.

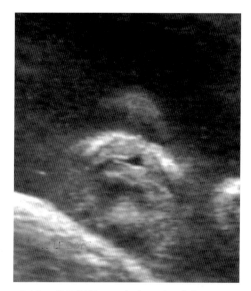

Figure 6.36 CHARGE association: the cleft.

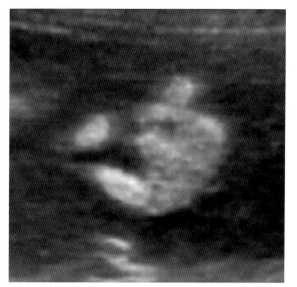

Figure 6.37 CHARGE association: the abnormal ear.

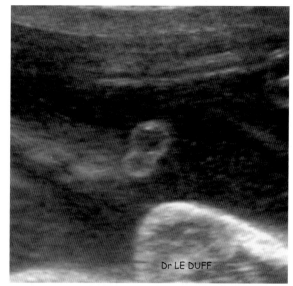

Figure 6.38 CHARGE association: hydramnios with UUA.

The verification of the presence of the upper semicircular canals[15] is possible during morphological US at a gestational age of 22 weeks, on a plane that is close to that of the biparietal diameter (Fig. 6.39). The upper canals appear as two small echogenic lines situated a third posterior to the insertion of the tentorium cerebelli (Figs 6.39 and 6.40). Another different view allows us to visualize the three canals (Fig. 6.41); however, this becomes impossible by the third trimester due to the ossification of the petrous part of the temporal bone.

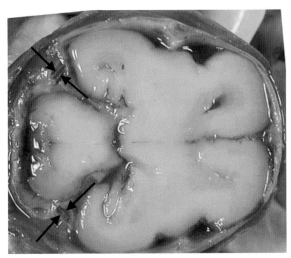

Figure 6.39 Macroscopic view of the upper semicircular canal (arrows).

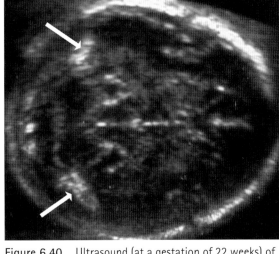

Figure 6.40 Ultrasound (at a gestation of 22 weeks) of the upper semicircular canal (arrows).

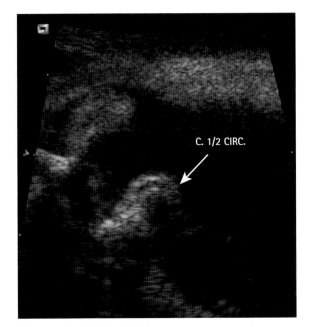

Figure 6.41 Another incidence of the semicircular canal.

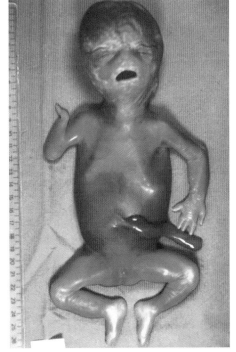

Figure 6.42 External view of Cornelia de Lange's syndrome.

Cornelia de Lange's syndrome[16]

This syndrome—also called de Lange's syndrome or Brachmann–de Lange syndrome—should be considered if there are limb anomalies of the first order (Fig. 6.42) (going from an oligodactyly to a phocomely). The most characteristic element, dysmorphism with synophrys, is not detectable by US. We must nonetheless consider this syndrome when faced with the association of IURG with hypogenitalism and anomalies of the limb especially in the cubital ray.

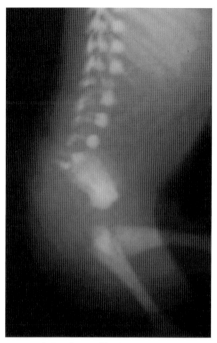

Figure 6.43 Spine in profile showing the straightness and shortness of the sacrum in a VACTERL association with an imperforate anus.

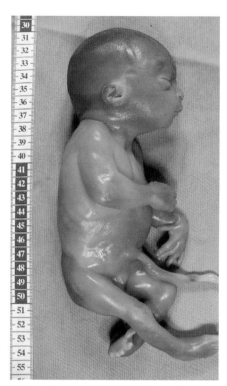

Figure 6.44 Fetus with VACTERL. Note the deformations of Potter's facies that resulted from the lack of amniotic fluid due to renal agenesis.

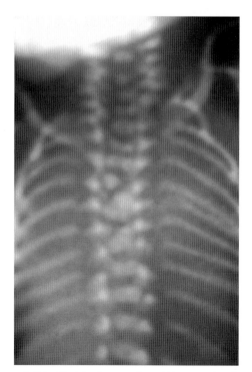

Figure 6.45 Vertebral anomalies at the same level as a tracheo–esophageal (T–E) fistula.

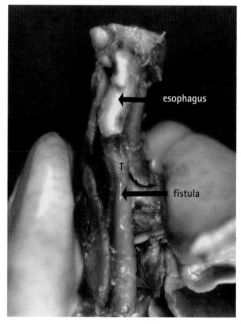

Figure 6.46 Posterior view of a HLB with a T–E fistula.

Cardiopathies associated with skeletal anomalies

In carefully examining the spine, all the way to the sacrum (Fig. 6.43), the straightness and/or short-ness of the lumbosacral spine could be an indirect sign of an anal imperforation. This crippling patho-logy is one of the key elements in the VACTERL association (Fig. 6.44).[18] This acronym stands for the association of at least three of the following components:

Vertebral anomalies (hemivertebrae—Fig. 6.45— and, at the same level, esophageal atresia and/ or a sacrum anomaly)

Anal imperforation

Cardiac anomalies

Tracheo–esophageal (T–E) fistula with the upper part of esopahgus (Fig. 6.46; see also Fig. 6.9), which is responsible for a variable excess of amniotic fluid

Esophageal atresia

Radial aplasia or **R**enal anomalies

Limb anomalies (when "R" illustrates the renal anomaly).

This association, where cardiopathy presents in al-most 50% of cases,[19] is generally sporadic. It appears to be AR when associated with a ventricular dila-tation, which is why examining the cephalic pole is extremely important here.

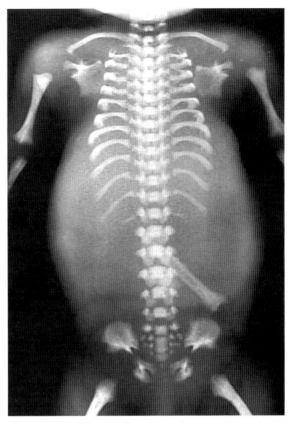

Figure 6.47   Ellis–van Creveld syndrome: radiography showing short long bones and ribs.

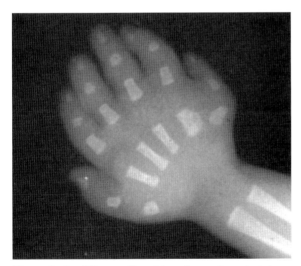

Figure 6.48   Ellis–van Creveld syndrome: hexadactyly.

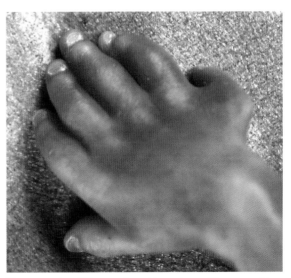

Figure 6.49   Ellis–van Creveld syndrome (the same fetus as in Figure 6.48): hexadactyly.

Long bones

Certain chondrodysplasias are associated with cardiopathies. The biometry of the long bones, and the aspect of the ribs should be examined with care because any bone impairment can be both late and discrete. In Ellis–van Creveld syndrome (Fig. 6.47), the cardiopathy, which often takes the form of a UA with an AVSD, could perhaps be primary. We look for hexadactyly (Figs 6.48 and 6.49), which is present in this syndrome. Several cases of LIAVV without defects, a minor form of AVSD, have been described in currently unpublished studies of the different forms of chondrodysplasia.

The study of the limbs and extremities is of the utmost importance. Certain major forms, such as complete aplasias of the radial ray, certain VACTERL association anomalies, or major anomalies in certain syndromes such as Cornelia de Lange's could be detected early. In these cases, the most subtle forms will remain difficult to discern if we do not rigorously attempt to visualize the two hands open counting all five fingers per hand. The frequent hexadactyly in SLOS, which is practically a constant in Ellis–van Creveld syndrome, should suggest a syndrome diagnosis when discovered in the fetal–pathologic examination.

Cardiopathies associated with cephalic anomalies

The appreciation of a fetal dysmorphia, key to a pediatric diagnosis, is unclear in classic US; 3D US now opens new perspectives in this field. Using US, we first begin by examining the following:

- Profile. The nasal bones (FNB),[20] their shortness (normal is 7 mm at 22 gestational weeks) is a warning; their absence is suspicious, testifying to a dysmorphic rule. A retrognathism is often an indirect sign of a cleft palate which we must try to confirm (Figs 6.50 and 6.51). It is often difficult to define the impression of dysmorphia explicitly, but we must try to refine this description. (One example would be the philtrum of fetal alcohol syndrome, where the mental prognosis is so negative.)
- Researching an atresia choanae (the "A" in CHARGE) which can be seen simply by looking for transnasal flow on Doppler imaging in the context of hydramnios.
- Face. Investigation of a labial cleft, often associated with a cardiopathy.
- Biparietal diameter views and sagittal views of the brain should allow us to perform the most

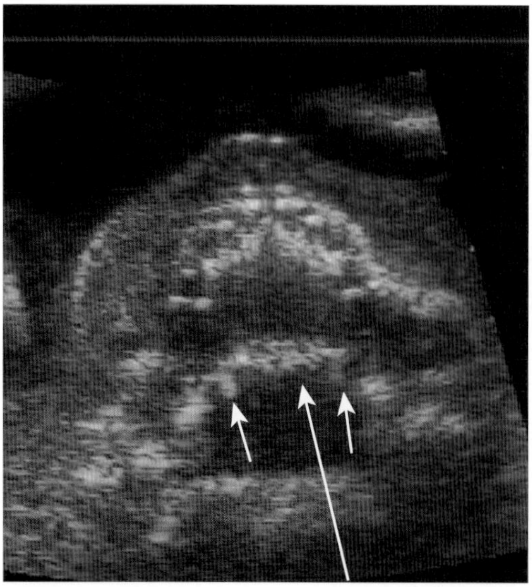

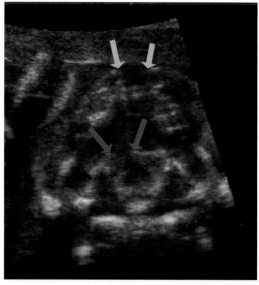

Figure 6.50   Normal palate.

Figure 6.51   Labio-duplication (green arrows) of the uvula (red arrows) in complete cleft palate.

complete possible cerebral assessment. Here we systematically investigate for a corpus callosum pathology, cerebellar vermix, or indirect signs of defaults in the closing of the neural tube. These are investigated, especially in VACTERL, in order to find if there is a dilatation of the ventricle. This association, considered sporadic, is in fact AR in cases associated with VACTERL with hydrocephaly.

- Verification of the semicircular canals (see above).
- Examination of the ears becomes more pertinent in 3D when we understand the importance of this examination in light of a facial dysmorphia. An example is the constant asymmetry of the ears in the CHARGE association (see Fig. 6.37).[15]

Cardiopathy associated with visceral anomalies

We should think of a visceroatrial heterotaxia (VAH) when faced with a situs anomaly associated with a complex cardiopathy with a normal karyotype, but also when there are signs of minor cardiac problems. If this has not already been done, it is important to verify the position of the abdominal organs diligently (median liver, the stomach). In this family of VAH, the situs is variable.[21] It is rarely recognized, in the case of a complete situs inversus, if we do not systematically verify the laterality when the stomach and the apex are on the same side. The cardiopathy is often complex, and associated with anomalies of the pulmonary or systemic venous return, a unique atrium, an AVSD or a unique ventricle with transposed vessels, and a PA with OS. We must examine with care the abdominal and thoracic vessels looking for the absence of IVC and azygous venous return (a left isomerism), or a TAPVR (a right isomerism).

A diaphragmatic hernia with the presence of intrathoracic abdominal viscera should lead us to look for other signs associated with Fryns' syndrome. The IURG is often late, but the distal phalanges are always short, and facial dysmorphia is considered where there is a cleft and/or the absence of FNB. In Cornelia de Lange's syndrome, on the other hand, the anomalies of the superior limbs (more affecting the cubital ray), like the wings of a bird, are easier to find than a dysmorphia.

On the level of the digestive tubes, the anomalies are understood through signs that are more indirect. A stomach can be poorly visualized, or not visualized at all in the case of a T–E fistula. Now, certain techniques allow the US diagnosis of atresia of the esophagus (see Figs 6.9 and 6.46) and the fistula.

At the level of the kidneys an oligoamnios, which can often evolve into an anamnios, hampers the examination of the heart and other organs. This should lead us to consider renal malformations (after verification of the absence of a 22 q11 deletion) which are frequent conditions of polymalformation syndromes.

The external genital organ examination (EGO) is of particular interest. In syndrome pathologies, the EGO, especially in male fetuses, can show a hypoplasia in CHARGE or discordance, i.e. hypoplasia, even feminine (see Fig. 6.32), in a fetus with 46XY in SLOS, and in Cornelia de Lange's syndrome.

> The verification of the architecture of the fetal heart—the primary objective of the US specialist—should always be completed by an attentive and thorough verification of the fetal morphology. It is crucial to do everything necessary to eliminate—as much as possible—the risk of associated malformations before sending the fetus affected by a cardiopathy to the pediatric cardiology team.

References

1. Cicero S, Sacchini C, Rembouskos G, Nicolaides KH. Sonographic markers of fetal aneuploidy—a review. Placenta 2003; 24 (suppl B):S88–S98.
2. Tennstedt C, Chaoui R, Körner H, Dietel M. Spectrum of congenital heart defects and extracardiac malformations associated with chromosomal abnormalities: results of a seven-year necropsy study. Heart 1999; 82(1):34–39.
3. Fredouille C, Piercecchi-Marti MD, Liprandi A et al. Linear insertion of atrioventricular valves without septal defect: a new anatomical landmark for Down's syndrome?

Fetal Diagn Ther 2002; 17(3):188–192. Erratum in: Fetal Diagn Ther 2002; 17(5):292.

4. Fredouille C, Baschet N, Morice JE et al. Linear insertion of the atrioventricular valves without defect. Arch Mal Coeur Vaiss 2005; 98(5):549–555. In French.

5. Viossat P, Cans C, Marchal-André D et al. Role of "subtle" ultrasonographic signs during antenatal screening for trisomy 21 during the second trimester of pregnancy: meta-analysis and CPDPN protocol of the Grenoble University Hospital. J Gynecol Obstet Biol Reprod (Paris) 2005; 34(3 Pt 1):215–231. In French.

6. Moyano D, Huggon IC, Allan LD. Fetal echocardiography in trisomy 18. Arch Dis Child Fetal Neonatal Ed 2005; 90(6):F520–F522; epub May 24, 2005.

7. Souka AP, von Kaisenberg CS, Hyett JA et al. Increased nuchal translucency with normal karyotype Am J Obstet Gynecol 2005; 192(4):1005–1021. Erratum in: Am J Obstet Gynecol 2005; 192(6):2096.

8. Boudjemline Y, Fermont L, Le Bidois J et al. Prevalence of 22q11 deletion in fetuses with conotruncal cardiac defects: a 6-year prospective study. J Pediatr 2001; 138(4):520–524.

9. Chaoui R, Kalache KD, Heling KS et al. Absent or hypoplastic thymus on ultrasound: a marker for deletion 22q11.2 in fetal cardiac defects. Ultrasound Obstet Gynecol 2002; 20(6):546–552.

10. Maymon R, Weinraub Z, Herman A. Pregnancy outcome of euploid fetuses with increased nuchal translucency: how bad is the news? J Perinat Med 2005; 33(3):191–198.

11. Carmichael SL, Shaw GM, Yang W, Lammer EJ. Maternal periconceptional alcohol consumption and risk for conotruncal heart defects. Birth Defects Res A Clin Mol Teratol 2003; 67(10):875–878.

12. Goldenberg A, Wolf C, Chevy F et al. Antenatal manifestations of Smith–Lemli–Opitz (RSH) syndrome: a retrospective survey of 30 cases. Am J Med Genet A 2004; 124(4):423–426.

13. Shackleton CH, Roitman E, Kratz L, Kelley R. Dehydro-oestriol and dehydropregnanetriol are candidate analytes for prenatal diagnosis of Smith–Lemli–Opitz syndrome. Prenat Diagn 2001; 21(3):207–212.

14. Sanlaville D, Etchevers HC, Gonzales M et al. Phenotypic spectrum of CHARGE syndrome in fetuses with CHD7 truncating mutations correlates with expression during human development. J Med Genet 2006; 43(3):211–317; epub Sep 16, 2005.

15. Verloes A. Updated diagnostic criteria for CHARGE syndrome: a proposal. Am J Med Genet A 2005; 133(3):306–308.

16. Greenwood RD, Sommer A, Craenen J et al. Congenital heart disease in de Lange's syndrome. South Med J 1977; 70(1):80–81.

17. Mehta AV, Ambalavanan SK. Occurrence of congenital heart disease in children with Brachmann–de Lange syndrome. Am J Med Genet 1997; 71(4):434–435.

18. Botto LD, Khoury MJ, Mastroiacovo P et al. The spectrum of congenital anomalies of the VATER association: an international study. Am J Med Genet 1997; 71(1):8–15.

19. Stoll C, Garne E, Clementi M for the EUROSCAN Study Group. Evaluation of prenatal diagnosis of associated congenital heart diseases by fetal ultrasonographic examination in Europe. Prenat Diagn 2001 21(4):243–252.

20. Bourlière-Najean B, Russel AS, Panuel M et al. Value of fetal skeletal radiographs in the diagnosis of fetal death. Eur Radiol 2003; 13(5):1046–1049; epub Jul 4, 2002.

21. Machado-Atias I, Anselmi G, Machado-Hernandez I, Febres C. Discordances between the different types of atrial arrangement and the positions of the thoracic–abdominal organs. Cardiol Young 2001 11(5):543–550.

Chapter 7

Points to remember

by Catherine Fredouille and Jean-Eric Develay-Morice

In order to examine the fetal heart efficiently, certain rules must be followed.

TECHNICAL POINTS TO REMEMBER

The technical rules for obtaining an excellent image are:

- An ideal exposition in the zone of interest due to:
  - appropriate windows to the fetal position
  - a perpendicular approach to the zones of interest
  - an extensive use of the zoom, but also:
- An optimal use of settings with:
  - a specific pre-adjustment, specifically for the heart
  - a constant modification of the gain
  - appropriate focal zones.

The use of Doppler, which is limited to certain indications, imposes the use of a "box" of minimal size.

Throughout our examination we acquire—and pay special attention in choosing—the highest quality images. After the examination, these will stand as proof of normality or pathology of the heart, even when interpreted by other operators and specialists.

KEY POINTS TO REMEMBER

By understanding ultrasound settings (US) we can use them to our advantage. By their correct use, with constant attention to acquiring excellent views, we can avoid many of the pitfalls we are confronted with in these examinations. Thus while acquiring our views we can use the three steps and ten key points methodology to verify if a fetal heart is normal or not.

The **first step** verifies position with:

- **Point 1:** laterality and position of the organs and vessels.
- **Point 2:** the axis of the heart should normally be at an angle of around 45°.

This is determined by carrying out the "elevator" from the TAD to the "optimal" four-chamber view along two vessels, the aorta and the IVC.

The **second step** verifies the inlet and is only accomplished using the "optimal" four-chamber view defined by three reference marks: the apex and the two inferior pulmonary veins (PVs). The presence of one or two complete ribs, depending on the approach of the view, allows us to ensure the axis of the image.

The following must appear in this view:

- **Point 3:** the heart, with its apex to the left, is attached to the lungs by the two inferior PVs.
- **Point 4:** there are four chambers.
- **Point 5:** contractile, balanced, and concordant.
- **Point 6:** the crux of the heart should show an offsetting of the atrioventricular valves.

The **third step** verifies the outlet and necessitates several complementary views to allow us to visualize:

- **Point 7:** two outlet chambers separated by an aligned outlet septum.
- **Point 8:** two conjoined vessels which cross over and are superimposed.
- **Point 9:** balanced and concordant outflow tracts.
- **Point 10:** a hooked arch arising at the center of the heart and giving rise to the three vessels of the neck.

The examination of the fetal heart begins at the level of the TAD view and goes up through the "elevator" towards the "optimal" four-chamber view.

You must verify that:

- The stomach, the aorta, and the apex of the heart are on the same *left* side.
- The *axis* of the heart is at an angle of around 45°.
- The outlet vessels must be balanced (in pathology, if one, for instance has a large diameter, the other will have a small one).

PATHOLOGIES TO REMEMBER

Through this method, the discovery of a pathology allows us to "classify" it into one of the different families and thus place it into the context of its associated pathologies or complications.

The position anomalies

Position anomalies are more frequently related to the visceroatrial heterotaxias, which have a normal karyotype.

The inlet anomalies

Depending on the anomaly, we observe:

- The pathologies of symmetry: a hypoplastic LV is more frequent than a hypoplastic RV, tricuspid atresia, and Ebstein's disease.
- The pathologies of the AVSD spectrum mainly touch the crux of the heart, one of the major warning signs of trisomy 21, but of other pathologies as well.

Outlet anomalies

Outlet anomalies fall into to two principal categories:

- Complete transposition of the great vessels, as a rule seen in isolation in an otherwise normal fetus. *This is one of the most important diagnoses not to overlook.*
- Frequent conotruncal cardiopathies (CTCs). These are present in numerous chromosomal anomalies, but also in polymalformation syndromes. We know of the preferred relationship that certain CTCs have with 22q11 chromosomal deletion (IAA, or PA with OS, and MAPCA).

In these pathologies of inlet and outlet, there can exist (at the same time) flow anomalies which translate into asymmetries in the size of the chambers or the diameters of the great vessels.

MORPHOLOGICAL POINTS TO REMEMBER

The morphological examination should be complete, but still oriented by the type of cardiopathy or the gravity of certain syndromes. Certain associated elements such as IURG, amniotic fluid anomalies (oligo- or hydramnios), and malformations of the face or extremities should make us very cautious.

Investigating for certain particular anomalies should be attempted, for instance in the case of semicircular canals, an important element of the CHARGE association, which is sometimes identifiable by the second trimester.

The right course to take varies depending on what we are faced with. The prognosis can be poor when criteria for polymalformation are found even when associated with minor cardiopathy. The outcome is very different when we see a more serious cardiopathy, but where the fetus is found to have a known normal karyotype and a totally reassuring extracardiac US examination.

In the absence of *all* associated pathologies detectable by systematic karyotype (with a research into 22q11 deletion for CTC), including the detailed morphological study, the precise diagnosis of the type of cardiopathy and its prognosis becomes essential and is the priority. This then becomes the domain of the pediatric cardiology team.

Any isolated cardiopathy will be given to the pediatric cardiologist to make a precise diagnosis and prognosis which will guide the pre-, per-, and postnatal approach.

Because of legislation and the advice of a multidisciplinary center for prenatal diagnosis combined with parental wishes, a medical termination of pregnancy might be proposed when we are faced with certain polymalformations or complex cardiopathies that offer *no* hope.

Faced with a curable cardiopathy, the pediatric cardiology team takes charge of the follow-up of the patient at birth.

CONCLUSION

Throughout this book our goal has been to approach the examination of the fetal heart in a simple and practical way. This will allow ultrasound specialists and operators to perform these examination with less apprehension and more confidence. Moreover it will ensure the best possible performance and the clearest, most interpretable results.

We only find what we look for.

We only look for what we know.

We only know what we understand.

Index

Abbreviations used in the index can be found on pages xv–xvi.
Page references in *italics* refer to figures.

ELSEVIER DVD-VIDEO LICENCE AGREEMENT

TERM This Agreement will remain in effect until terminated pursuant to the terms of this Agreement. You may terminate this Agreement at any time by removing from Your system and destroying the Product and any copies of the Proprietary Material. Unauthorized copying of the Product, including without limitation, the Proprietary Material and documentation, or otherwise failing to comply with the terms and conditions of this Agreement shall result in automatic termination of this licence and will make available to Elsevier legal remedies. Upon termination of this Agreement, the licence granted herein will terminate and You must immediately destroy the Product and all copies of the Product and of the Proprietary Material, together with any and all accompanying documentation. All provisions relating to proprietary rights shall survive termination of this Agreement.

LIMITED WARRANTY AND LIMITATION OF LIABILITY Elsevier warrants that the software embodied in this Product will perform in substantial compliance with the documentation supplied in this Product, unless the performance problems are the result of hardware failure or improper use. If You report a significant defect in performance in writing to Elsevier within ninety (90) calendar days of your having purchased the Product, and Elsevier is not able to correct same within sixty (60) days after its receipt of Your notification, You may return this Product, including all copies and documentation, to Elsevier and Elsevier will refund Your money. In order to apply for a refund on your purchased Product, please contact the return address on the invoice to obtain the refund request form ("Refund Request Form"), and either fax or mail your signed request and your proof of purchase to the address indicated on the Refund Request Form. Incomplete forms will not be processed. Defined terms in the Refund Request Form shall have the same meaning as in this Agreement.

YOU UNDERSTAND THAT, EXCEPT FOR THE LIMITED WARRANTY RECITED ABOVE, ELSEVIER, ITS AFFILIATES, LICENSORS, THIRD PARTY SUPPLIERS AND AGENTS (TOGETHER "THE SUPPLIERS") MAKE NO REPRESENTATIONS OR WARRANTIES, WITH RESPECT TO THE PRODUCT, INCLUDING, WITHOUT LIMITATION THE PROPRIETARY MATERIAL. ALL OTHER REPRESENTATIONS, WARRANTIES, CONDITIONS OR OTHER TERMS, WHETHER EXPRESS OR IMPLIED BY STATUTE OR COMMON LAW, ARE HEREBY EXCLUDED TO THE FULLEST EXTENT PERMITTED BY LAW.

IN PARTICULAR BUT WITHOUT LIMITATION TO THE FOREGOING NONE OF THE SUPPLIERS MAKE ANY REPRESENTATIONS OR WARRANTIES (WHETHER EXPRESS OR IMPLIED) REGARDING THE PERFORMANCE OF YOUR PAD, NETWORK OR COMPUTER SYSTEM WHEN USED IN CONJUNCTION WITH THE PRODUCT, NOR THAT THE PRODUCT WILL MEET YOUR REQUIREMENTS OR THAT ITS OPERATION WILL BE UNINTERRUPTED OR ERROR-FREE.

EXCEPT IN RESPECT OF DEATH OR PERSONAL INJURY CAUSED BY THE SUPPLIERS' NEGLIGENCE AND TO THE FULLEST EXTENT PERMITTED BY LAW, IN NO EVENT (AND REGARDLESS OF WHETHER SUCH DAMAGES ARE FORESEEABLE AND OF WHETHER SUCH LIABILITY IS BASED IN TORT, CONTRACT OR OTHERWISE) WILL ANY OF THE SUPPLIERS BE LIABLE TO YOU FOR ANY DAMAGES (INCLUDING, WITHOUT LIMITATION, ANY LOST PROFITS, LOST SAVINGS OR OTHER SPECIAL, INDIRECT, INCIDENTAL OR CONSEQUENTIAL DAMAGES ARISING OUT OF OR RESULTING FROM: (I) YOUR USE OF, OR INABILITY TO USE, THE PRODUCT; (II) DATA LOSS OR CORRUPTION; AND/OR (III) ERRORS OR OMISSIONS IN THE PROPRIETARY MATERIAL.

IF THE FOREGOING LIMITATION IS HELD TO BE UNENFORCEABLE, OUR MAXIMUM LIABILITY TO YOU IN RESPECT THEREOF SHALL NOT EXCEED THE AMOUNT OF THE LICENCE FEE PAID BY YOU FOR THE PRODUCT. THE REMEDIES AVAILABLE TO YOU AGAINST ELSEVIER AND THE LICENSORS OF MATERIALS INCLUDED IN THE PRODUCT ARE EXCLUSIVE.

If the information provided In the Product contains medical or health sciences information, it is intended for professional use within the medical field. Information about medical treatment or drug dosages is intended strictly for professional use, and because of rapid advances in the medical sciences, independent verification of diagnosis and drug dosages should be made. The provisions of this Agreement shall be severable, and in the event that any provision of this Agreement is found to be legally unenforceable, such unenforceability shall not prevent the enforcement or any other provision of this Agreement.

GOVERNING LAW This Agreement shall be governed by the laws of England and Wales. In any dispute arising out of this Agreement, you and Elsevier each consent to the exclusive personal jurisdiction and venue in the courts of England and Wales.

DVD PLAYER ACCESS INSTRUCTIONS

- Place the DVD in the DVD player and press play. Use the up and down arrows on your remote control to navigate the menus. Press **Enter** or **Play** to make a selection.

DVD-ROM ACCESS INSTRUCTIONS

- Locate the DVD icon in **My Computer** or select "**Start**", "**Programs**" and the name of the DVD software
- Click the DVD icon or the name of the DVD software and the **Main Menu** will appear.
- Macintosh users can simply double-click the DVD icon.

SYSTEM REQUIREMENTS

Windows PC
PC Based Pentium 450MHZ
Windows 98/98SE, ME, 2000, NT 4.0 Service Pack 6 (SP6) or higher
256MB RAM or higher
32 MB or higher Graphics Card
4X DVD-ROM drive
Display Resolution of 800x600 or greater
Sound Card and Speakers
Software which supports DVD-Video playback

Macintosh
Power PC G3 300MHZ, I-MAC, I-Book
Macintosh OS 9.2 or higher
256MB RAM or higher
32 MB or higher Graphics Card
4X DVD-ROM drive
Display Resolution of 800x600 or greater
Sound Card and Speakers
Software which supports DVD-Video playback

Technical support for this product is available between 7.30 a.m. and 7.00 p.m. CST,
Monday through Friday.
Before calling, be sure that your computer meets the minimum system requirements to run this software.
Inside the United States and Canada, call 1-800-692-9010.
Inside the United Kingdom, call 0-0800-6929-0100.
Rest of World, call +1-314-872-8370.
You may also fax your questions to +1-314-523-4932,
or contact Technical Support through e-mail: technical.support@elsevier.com.